Color Atlas
and
Synopsis of
Clinical Dermatology

Thomas B. Fitzpatrick, M.D., Ph.D., D.Sc. (Hon.)
Wigglesworth Professor of Dermatology
Harvard Medical School
Dermatologist
Massachusetts General Hospital
Consultant in Dermatology
Brigham and Women's Hospital,
The Children's Hospital, and Beth Israel Hospital
Boston, Massachusetts

Machiel K. Polano, M.D.
Emeritus Professor and Chairman
Department of Dermatology
University Hospital
Leiden, The Netherlands

Dick Suurmond, M.D.
Professor and Chairman
Department of Dermatology
University Hospital
Leiden, The Netherlands

Richard Allen Johnson, M.D.C.M.
Clinical Instructor in Dermatology
Harvard Medical School
Clinical Associate in Dermatology
Massachusetts General Hospital
Associate in Dermatology
Beth Israel Hospital
Associate Physician (Dermatology)
Brigham and Women's Hospital
Boston, Massachusetts

McGraw-Hill Information Services Company
HEALTH PROFESSIONS DIVISION

New York   St. Louis   San Francisco   Colorado Springs   Auckland   Bogotá   Hamburg
Lisbon   London   Madrid   Mexico   Milan   Montreal   New Delhi   Panama   Paris   San Juan
São Paulo   Singapore   Sydney   Tokyo   Toronto

FIRST PRINTING: DECEMBER 1982

Updated and Reprinted: December 1983, October 1984, September 1985, August 1986, July 1987, May 1988, January 1989

Color Atlas and Synopsis of Clinical Dermatology

89LEHHOR89432109

ISBN 0-07-021197-3

This book was set in Helvetica by York Graphic Services, Inc.; the editors were Robert P. McGraw, Donna McIvor, and Steven Tenney; the production supervisor was Jeanne Skahan; the designer was Murray Fleminger.

The printer was Lehigh Press Lithographers; the binder, A. Horowitz & Son Bookbinders.

Library of Congress Cataloging in Publication Data

Fitzpatrick, Thomas B.
  Color atlas and synopsis of clinical dermatology.

  1. Skin—Diseases—Atlases. I. Polano, Machiel K.
II. Suurmond, Dick. III. Title. [DNLM:
1. Dermatology—Atlases. 2. Skin diseases. WR 17
F559c]
RL81.F58 1983   616.5   82-17080
ISBN 0-07-021197-3

The color photographs herein were done by H. Korff and J. v.d. Walle of the Audiovisual Service of the Medical Faculty in Leiden, The Netherlands, and are from the collection of the Department of Dermatology, University Medical Centre, Leiden. The color plates were prepared in the lithographic institute Sturm of Basel, Switzerland, on appointment by CIBA-GEIGY, Basel. The superb cooperation of CIBA-GEIGY is gratefully acknowledged.

Contents

XIX. Dermatologic Artifacts (Factitial Dermatitis)

Appendices

Index of Differential Diagnosis by Regions

Subject Index

Preface
to the Eighth Printing

What's the use of a book,"
thought Alice,
"without pictures or conversations?"

Lewis Carroll
Alice's Adventures in Wonderland

For an increasing number of physicians who are not dermatologists, the management of skin disorders has recently become a major challenge. This is because of changes in the practice of medicine in which referral to specialists is being severely restricted by third-party insurance carriers. Familiarity with dermatology is necessary because of the large number of patients presenting with skin lesions as incidental findings or major complaints that are now being seen first by the primary care physician, pediatrician, and certain types of internists (allergists, rheumatologists, infectious disease consultants). The prevalence of skin lesions and skin disorders now extant has stimulated general physicians to become "paraspecialists" in dermatology. Just as a chest physician must look at and interpret the chest film or the orthopedist the bone films, so the nondermatologist must now be able to "read" skin lesions, as he or she should be able to interpret a blood smear. There are skin markers of multisystem disease that are discovered in well people; these are important because if these lesions are overlooked, the patient's future health may be in jeopardy and, furthermore, there are medical-legal implications. Certain skin lesions are as important to discover as palpable lymph nodes (e.g., early malignant melanoma, hyperlipoproteinemic xanthomas, cutaneous T-cell lymphoma, erythema nodosum, and skin signs of AIDS).

This atlas-text has a single and specific goal: to acquaint the physician with the principal lesions of the skin in order to facilitate dermatologic diagnosis. Correct therapy is based on correct diagnosis. Inasmuch as dermatologic lesions are visually identified, the logical approach to learning how to make a dermatologic diagnosis is first and foremost to carefully study a color illustration of typical lesions and, simultaneously, while viewing the lesions, to read a succinct summary of the major features of the disease. With this aim in mind, we have juxtaposed large color photographs of skin lesions opposite a one-page synopsis of the essential facts of diagnosis and treatment of all the ten groups of the most prevalent skin disorders.

The text of this atlas was a cooperative effort between Leiden (The Netherlands) and Boston (United States). The case histories were done by M. K. Polano and D. Suurmond, and the therapeutic modalities reflect their practices; the disease summaries, approaches, drawings, and appendices were done by T. B. Fitzpatrick; a vigorous discussion among the three authors resulted in the final text. The color plates are from the collection of the Department of Dermatology, University Medical Centre, Leiden, The Netherlands. Photographs were taken by Hans Korff and J. v. d. Walle. The color plates were prepared in the lithographic institute Sturm of Basel, Switzerland, on appointment by CIBA-GEIGY, Basel. We are grateful to CIBA-GEIGY for their permission to use them in this book.

The line drawings and halftones were prepared by Gail Burroughs except for the three halftones depicting primary melanoma, which were done by Gail Cooper.

The authors are grateful to Patricia K. Novak for the preparation of the manuscript. Beatrice Fitzpatrick read the manuscript for clarity. The following colleagues read all or portions of the manuscript, and we are grateful to Drs. Jeffrey D. Bernhard,

Harley A. Haynes, Newton E. Hyslop, Jr., Arthur R. Rhodes, Nicholas A. Soter, Morton N. Swartz, and Robert S. Stern, all of the Harvard University Medical School.

Finally, we would like to cite the cooperation of Donna McIvor, Mariapaz R. Englis, Richard Laufer, and J. Dereck Jeffers of the McGraw-Hill Book Company.

Thomas B. Fitzpatrick
Machiel K. Polano
Dick Suurmond
Richard Allen Johnson

Acronyms

AIDS	acquired immunodeficiency syndrome
ANA	antinuclear antibody
ARC	AIDS-related complex
AST	antistreptolysin titer
BSR	blood sedimentation rate
ESR	erythrocyte sedimentation rate
FBS	fasting blood sugar
G-6-PD	glucose-6-phosphate dehydrogenase
HIV	human immunodeficiency virus
PAS	periodic acid Schiff
PMN	polymorphic neutrophilic leukocyte(s)
PUVA	psoralen plus ultraviolet A
RAST	radioallergosorbent test
RPR	rapid plasma reagin
SPF	sun protection factor
STS	serologic test for syphilis
TPI	*Treponema pallidum* immobilization
TSH	thyroid-stimulating hormone
UVA	ultraviolet radiation A (320–400 nm)
UVB	ultraviolet radiation B (300–320 nm)
VDRL	Venereal Disease Research Laboratory

Introduction

Approach to Diagnosis

The diagnosis of skin diseases or skin manifestations of multisystem diseases may be considered in four rather arbitrary approaches.

1. Single etiologic factor

    EXAMPLE *Urticaria from penicillin* (by history) or *tinea corporis* with demonstration of mycelia in skin scrapings (laboratory examination)

2. The skin lesions

    EXAMPLE *Acne:* comedo, papule, pustule, or cyst (physical examination only)

3. Pathophysiology—an altered physiologic response

    EXAMPLE *Cold urticaria,* the lesions being induced by application of ice to the skin with the development of an urticarial wheal

4. Syndrome or reaction pattern to multiple etiologies

    EXAMPLE *Porphyria cutanea tarda:* bullae or erosions, pink scars on dorsa of the hands, hirsutism, elevated uroporphyrin levels in the urine (laboratory), related to ingestion of ethanol or estrogens
    Necrotizing vasculitis: palpable purpura on lower third of legs (physical examination), arthralgia, abdominal pain, peripheral neuritis (history), elevated erythrocyte sedimentation rate, reduced serum complement, red cell casts, biopsy showing fibrinoid deposits in walls of venules, extravasation of erythrocytes (laboratory examination), related to drugs, infections, collagen-vascular disease, or lymphoma

The task is to make the diagnosis by a methodical approach using a checklist that facilitates the aggregation of the facts: history, physical examination (skin lesions, miscellaneous noncutaneous physical findings), dermatopathology, and other laboratory and special examinations. The Outline of an Approach to Dermatologic Diagnosis is an attempt to fulfill this need.

How should the beginner approach dermatology?

First, one should be thoroughly familiar with the "bumps and blemishes" (the background noise) that may be encountered in the general physical examination (see inside back cover for these lesions and diseases).

Second, the physician should carefully study the photographs and thoroughly read the précis of the four most prevalent diseases: acne, warts, eczema, and psoriasis.

Finally, one must become familiar with the six next most prevalent skin disorders: skin cancer, drug reactions, urticaria, and viral, bacterial, and mycotic infections.

With these guidelines you are off to a start—"Well begun is half done," said Friar Laurence in Shakespeare's *Romeo and Juliet.*

1

Outline of an Approach to Dermatologic Diagnosis

I. **Epidemiology and Etiology** (see Appendix A) Age, race, sex, occupation

II. **History**
   A. Duration of onset of skin lesions: days, weeks, months, years
   B. Relationship of skin lesions to season, heat, cold, previous treatment, drug ingestion, occupation, hobbies; effects of menses, pregnancy
   C. Skin symptoms: pruritus, pain, paresthesia
   D. Constitutional symptoms
      1. "Acute illness" syndrome: headache, chills, feverishness, weakness
      2. "Chronic illness" syndrome: fatigue, weakness, anorexia, weight loss, malaise
   E. Systems review

III. **Physical Examination**
   A. Appearance of patient: uncomfortable, "toxic," well
   B. Changes in body temperature: elevated
   C. Skin—four major skin signs: (1) type, (2) shape, (3) arrangement, (4) distribution of lesions

   1. **Type** of lesion (see Appendix B, pp 369–380)

Basic lesions	*Sequential lesions*
Macule	Scale
Papule-plaque	Exudation: dry (crust)
Wheal	wet (weeping)
Nodule	Erosion
Cyst	Scar
Vesicle-bulla	Lichenification
Pustule	
Ulcer (also sequential)	
Hyperkeratosis (also sequential)	
Sclerosis	
Atrophy (also sequential)	
Telangiectasia	
Infarct	
Purpura	

   Color of lesions or of the skin if diffuse involvement: *"skin color"; white:* leukoderma, hypomelanosis; *red:* erythema; *pink; violaceous; brown;* hypermelanosis; *black; blue; gray; orange; yellow.* Red or purple purpuric lesions do not blanch with pressure (diascopy).
   Palpation
      Consistency (soft, firm, hard, fluctuant, boardlike)
      Deviation in temperature (hot, cold)
      Mobility of lesion or of skin
      Presence of tenderness
      Estimate of the depth of lesion (i.e., dermal or subcutaneous)

   2. **Shape** of individual lesions
      Round, oval, polygonal, polycyclic, annular (ring-shaped), iris, serpiginous (snakelike), umbilicated

   3. **Arrangement** of multiple lesions
      Grouped: herpetiform, zosteriform, arciform, annular, reticulated (net-shaped), linear, serpiginous (snakelike)
      Disseminated: scattered discrete lesions or diffuse involvement (i.e., without identifiable borders)

    4. **Distribution** of lesions

       Extent: isolated (single lesion), localized, regional, generalized, universal

       Pattern: symmetrical, exposed areas, sites of pressure, intertriginous areas, follicular localization, random

       Characteristic patterns: scabies, secondary syphilis, psoriasis, seborrheic dermatitis, lichen planus, pityriasis rosea, dermatitis herpetiformis, atopic dermatitis, vitiligo, acne, erythema multiforme, candidiasis, contact dermatitis, lupus erythematosus, erythrasma, ichthyosis, pemphigus, pemphigoid, porphyria cutanea tarda, xanthoma, necrotizing angiitis (vasculitis)

D. Hair and nails

E. Mucous membranes

F. Miscellaneous physical findings: lymphadenopathy, hepatosplenomegaly, cardiac findings, neurologic findings (see Appendix E), ophthalmologic findings

IV. Differential Diagnosis

V. Laboratory and Special Examinations

A. Dermatopathology

    1. Light microscopy: site, process, cell types

    2. Immunofluorescence

    3. Special techniques: stains, electron microscopy, etc.

B. Microbiologic examination of skin specimens: scales, crusts, or exudate

    1. Direct microscopic examination of skin (see Appendix C)

       For yeast and fungus: 10% potassium hydroxide preparation (see pages 195, 201, 225, 381, 382, and Figure 74)

       For bacteria: Gram's stain

       For virus: Tzanck smear (see pages 242 and 382)

       For spirochetes: dark-field examination

       For parasites: scabies mite from a burrow (see page 382)

    2. Culture

       Bacterial ⎱
       Mycologic ⎰ For granulomas, culture of minced tissue

C. Laboratory examinations of blood

   Bacteriologic: culture

   Serologic: ANA, STS, serology

   Hematologic: hematocrit or hemoglobin, cells, differential smear

   Chemistry: fasting blood sugar, blood urea nitrogen, creatinine, liver function and thyroid function tests (if indicated)

D. Radiographic studies

E. Urinalysis

F. Stool examination (for occult blood, e.g., in vasculitis syndromes; for ova and parasites)

G. Wood's light examination (see page 381)

   Urine: pink-orange fluorescence in porphyria cutanea tarda (add 1.0 ml of 5.0% hydrochloric acid)

   Hair (in vivo): green fluorescence in tinea capitis (hair shaft)

   Skin (in vivo)

      Erythrasma: coral-red fluorescence

      Hypomelanosis: decrease in intensity

      Brown hypermelanosis: increase in intensity

      Blue hypermelanosis: no change in intensity

H. Patch testing (see page 381)

I. Acetowhitening—whitening of subclinical penile warts after application of 5% acetic acid (see page 236)

VI. Pathophysiology (see page 368)

VII. Course and Prognosis

VIII. Treatment

IX. General References

Arndt KA: *Manual of Dermatologic Therapeutics with Essentials of Diagnosis,* 4th ed, Little, Brown, Boston, 1989

Demis DJ et al (eds): *Clinical Dermatology,* 4 vol, Harper & Row, New York, 1979

Fitzpatrick TB et al (eds): *Dermatology in General Medicine,* 3d ed, 2 vol, McGraw-Hill, New York, 1987

Lever WF, Schaumburg-Lever G: *Histopathology of the Skin,* 6th ed. Lippincott, Philadelphia, 1983

Moschella SL, Hurley HJ Jr: *Dermatology,* 2d ed, 2 vol, Saunders, Philadelphia, 1985

Polano MK: *Topical Skin Therapeutics,* Churchill-Livingston, Edinburgh, 1984

Rook A et al (eds): *Textbook of Dermatology,* 4th ed, 3 vol, Blackwell, Oxford, 1986

I
Eczematous Dermatitis

Allergic Contact Dermatitis

Contact dermatitis is an acute, subacute, or chronic inflammation of the epidermis and dermis caused by external agents and characterized by pruritus or burning of the skin.

EPIDEMIOLOGY AND ETIOLOGY

Age No influence on capacity for sensitization

Race Black skin is less susceptible

Occupation This is the important cause of disability in industry.

Etiology Clinical syndrome usually *delayed-hypersensitivity reaction* (type IV) with a latent period of a few days or years from the first exposure and the reexposure that precipitates the allergic contact dermatitis, *or* a *primary* irritant which produces inflammation on first or repeated contact

HISTORY

Duration of Lesion(s) Acute contact— days, weeks; chronic contact—months, years

Skin Symptoms Pruritus

Constitutional Symptoms "Acute illness" syndrome (including fever) in severe allergic contact dermatitis (e.g., poison ivy)

PHYSICAL EXAMINATION

Skin Lesions

TYPE

Acute Irregular, poorly outlined patches of erythema and edema on which are superimposed closely spaced, nonumbilicated vesicles, punctate erosions exuding serum, and crusts

Subacute Patches of mild erythema showing small, dry scales or superficial desquamation, sometimes associated with small, red, pointed or rounded, firm papules

Chronic Patches of lichenification (thickening of the epidermis with deepening of the skin lines in parallel or rhomboidal pattern), with satellite, small, firm, rounded or flat-topped papules, excoriations, and pigmentation or mild erythema

ARRANGEMENT Often linear, with artificial patterns, an "outside job." Plant contact often results in linear lesions.

DISTRIBUTION

Extent Isolated, localized to one region (e.g., shoe dermatitis), or generalized (e.g., plant dermatitis)

Pattern Random or on exposed areas (as in airborne allergic contact or photocontact dermatitis)

Characteristic patterns See Figures I and II.

LABORATORY AND SPECIAL EXAMINATIONS

Dermatopathology Does not differentiate between allergic and primary irritant dermatitis

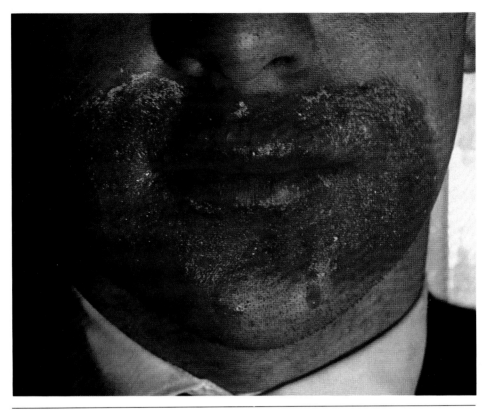

1 Contact eczematous dermatitis caused by balsam of Peru

Patient Profile *Twenty-year-old male student*

History *An itching eruption around the lips for 2 days; because of dry lips, the patient used a balsam-of-Peru–containing OTC preparation before the sudden appearance of this eruption.*

Physical Examination *Oval, sharply demarcated, erythematous, weeping, and scaling eruption*

Laboratory and Special Examinations *Patch test for contact sensitivity with balsam of Peru and the OTC preparations were strongly positive.*

Clues *Clinical aspect, history, and results of patch tests*

Treatment *Wet dressings and a bland cooling paste, followed by 1% hydrocortisone cream. The eruption disappeared in a few days.*

Significance *In order to avoid recurrences, the patient should not use substances giving cross-reactions with balsam of Peru, such as the essential oils of orange peel, cinnamon, and other spices.*

SITE Epidermis and dermis

PROCESS Inflammation with intraepidermal intercellular edema (spongiosis) and monocyte and histiocyte infiltration in the dermis suggest allergic contact dermatitis, while more superficial vesicles containing polymorphonuclear leukocytes suggest a primary irritant dermatitis. In chronic contact dermatitis there is lichenification (hyperkeratosis, acanthosis, elongation of rete ridges, and elongation and broadening of papillae).

PATCH TESTS Sensitization is present on every part of the skin; therefore application of the allergen to any area of normal skin will provoke inflammation. Patch tests should be delayed until the dermatitis has subsided at the selected site of application for at least 2 weeks. See page 381.

PATHOPHYSIOLOGY

Allergic contact dermatitis is the classic example of type IV hypersensitivity reaction (cellular, cell-mediated, delayed, or tuberculin type) caused by sensitized lymphocytes (T cells) after contact with antigen. The antigen processing can occur via Langerhans cells. The tissue damage results from cytotoxicity by T cells or from release of lymphokines.

TREATMENT

Acute Identify and remove the etiologic agent.

Vesicles may be drained but tops should not be removed.

Wet dressings using cloths soaked in Burrow's solution changed every 2 to 3 hr. Fourteen-day tapered course [70 mg on day 1 (14 5-mg tablets), taper by 1 tablet per day, divide daily dose into 3 doses at mealtime].

For severe generalized allergic contact dermatitis, prednisone is necessary.

Subacute and Chronic The newer superpotent topical corticosteroid preparations, betamethasone diproprionate and clobetasol proprionate, if not bullous.

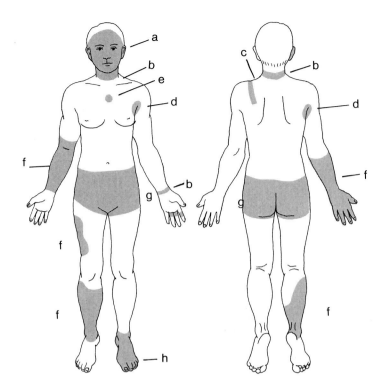

Figure I
Eczematous Dermatitis (Contact) (a) Airborne allergens (plants, pollens, sprays); (b) jewelry, clothing, furs; (c) clothing straps; (d) deodorant, antiperspirant; (e) metal tags; (f) plants; (g) trunks and panties; (h) shoes or hose.

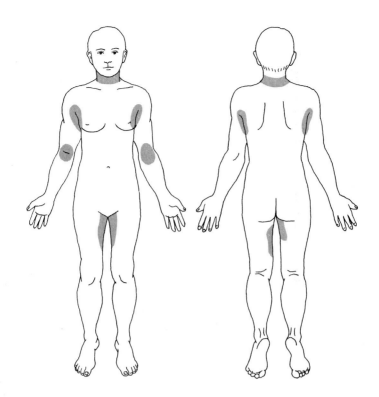

Figure II
Textile Dermatitis

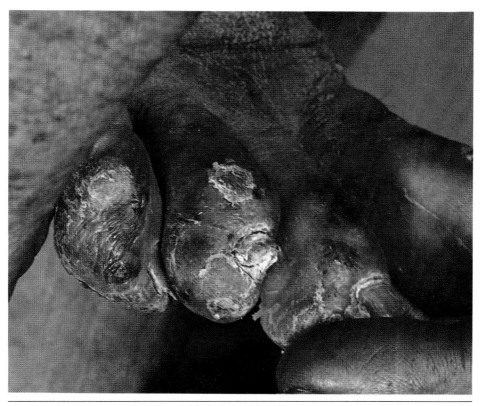

2 Contact eczematous dermatitis caused by shoes

Patient Profile Fifty-three-year-old female homemaker

History For 6 months, itching and scaling eruption of both feet, not responsive to various treatments

Physical Examination Circumscribed, red, oozing patches on the dorsa of toes III to V surrounded by scaling and redness. Scaling also on dorsa of feet. Interdigital spaces free.

Differential Diagnosis Dermatophytosis, contact dermatitis

Special Examinations Examination for fungi negative. Patch tests with 40 possible allergens that can be present in shoes: strongly positive on three different phenolformaldehyde-reactive resins and on pieces of the shoe.

Clues Localization on the dorsal and not on the intertriginous parts of the toes, and the result of patch tests

Significance The patient has in the future to avoid all shoes glued with reactive phenolformaldehyde resins.

Treatment Rapid improvement occurred after avoiding contact with shoes glued with the reactive phenolformaldehyde resins.

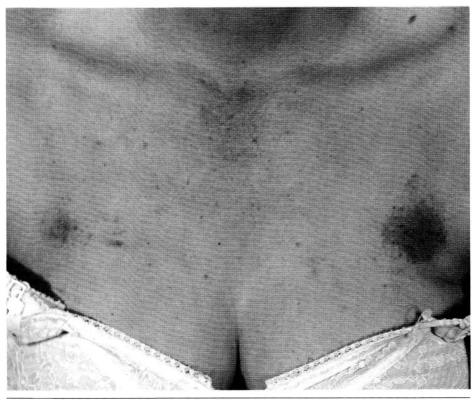

3 Contact eczematous dermatitis caused by nickel

Patient Profile Forty-two-year-old female homemaker

History For 6 months, two itching patches on the trunk above the breasts

Physical Examination Above the left breast, a sharply demarcated, erythematous, slightly infiltrated macule, surrounded by papules; above right breast, disseminated papules. Localization coincides with contact of buckles of the bra with the skin.

Special Examinations Patch tests for contact sensitivity: 5% nickel sulfate in water, strongly positive. Chrome: negative.

Clues Localization and patch test results

Treatment Replacement of the buckles by plastic buckles; 1% hydrocortisone cream

Significance In the future, patient has to avoid nickel in clothing apparel, watches, etc.

Atopic Dermatitis

Atopic dermatitis is an acute, subacute, but usually chronic, pruritic inflammation of the epidermis and dermis, often occurring in association with a personal or family history of hay fever, asthma, allergic rhinitis, or atopic dermatitis.

EPIDEMIOLOGY AND ETIOLOGY

Age Onset in first 2 months of life and by first year in 60 percent of patients

Sex Slightly more common in boys than girls

Hereditary Predisposition Over two-thirds have personal or family history of allergic rhinitis, hay fever, or asthma.

HISTORY

Duration of Lesions Most patients begin at age 2 to 12, and 60 percent by first year; 30 percent seen for the first time by age 5, with only 10 percent developing atopic dermatitis between 6 and 20 years of age. Mental stress is an important factor.

Skin Symptoms Pruritus is the sine qua non of atopic dermatitis. The constant scratching leads to a vicious cycle of itch-scratch-rash-itch—the rash being lichenification of the skin. Itching is precipitated by wool, a change in room temperature, and stress.

SKIN LESIONS

See Figures 4 to 7, Figure III.

SPECIAL CLINICAL FEATURES

Tendency to develop generalized infections, especially herpes simplex and vaccinia

White dermographism on stroking skin and/or delayed blanch to cholinergic agents

Anterior subcapsular cataracts in 10 percent, between 15 and 25 years of age

Infraorbital fold (Dennie-Morgan sign)

Infraorbital darkening

Facial pallor

Ichthyosis vulgaris in 10 percent of patients

DIFFERENTIAL DIAGNOSIS

Certain rare metabolic disorders mimic atopic dermatitis and these should be considered: acrodermatitis enteropathica, gluten-sensitive enteropathy, glucagonoma syndrome, histidinemia, phenylketonuria; also some immunologic disorders including Wiskott-Aldrich syndrome, sex-linked agammaglobulinemia, hyper-IgE syndrome, Letterer-Siwe disease, selective IgA deficiency.

DERMATOPATHOLOGY

Site Epidermis and dermis

Process Varying degrees of acanthosis with rare intraepidermal intercellular edema (spongiosis). The dermal infiltrate is comprised of lymphocytes, monocytes, and mast cells with few or no eosinophils.

LABORATORY EXAMINATION

Culture and sensitivity for bacterial infection

Culture for HSV if indicated

PATHOPHYSIOLOGY

Type I (IgE-mediated) hypersensitivity reaction occurring as a result of the release of vasoactive substances from both mast cells and basophils that have been sensitized by the interaction of the antigen with IgE (reaginic or skin-sensitizing antibody); however, the role of IgE in atopic dermatitis is still not clarified.

COURSE AND PROGNOSIS

Spontaneous incomplete remission during childhood is the rule with occasional, more severe recurrences during adolescence. In most patients the disease persists for 15 to 20 years. Disturbing is that 30 to 50 percent of patients will develop asthma or hay fever.

TREATMENT

Acute See page 8

Subacute and Chronic Atopic dermatitis is considered by many to be related, at least in part, to emotional stress. Allergic work-up is usually unrewarding in revealing an allergen (food, inhalant, etc.) and there is no benefit from immunotherapy. Oiled water baths and emollients are essential to prevent dryness of the skin which provokes itching and starts the cycle of itch-scratch-rash-itch. Soap should not be used. H_1 antihistamines are probably useful in reducing itching. Education of the patient to avoid rubbing and scratching is most important. Topical corticosteroids and crude coal-tar preparations are valuable agents but are useless if the patient continues to scratch and rub the plaques. Systemic corticosteroids should be avoided except in rare instances and for only short courses. Warn patients of their special problems with herpes simplex, and frequency of superimposed staphylococcal infection for which oral erythromycin is indicated and acyclovir if herpes simplex is suspected. Combinations of UVA and UVB phototherapy are helpful in chronic recalcitrant disease.

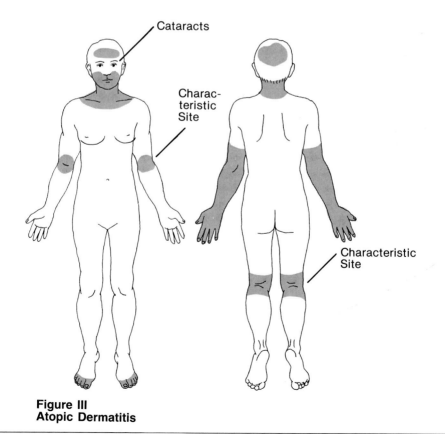

Cataracts

Charac-
teristic
Site

Characteristic
Site

Figure III
Atopic Dermatitis

Infantile Atopic Dermatitis

Infantile atopic dermatitis is one of the most troublesome skin eruptions in children. There is an "atopic" background without a clearly defined immunologic pattern. Skin lesions seem to be a reaction to itching and rubbing. Since the advent of topical corticosteroids, the problem has lost much of its seriousness.

PHYSICAL EXAMINATION

Skin Lesions

TYPE   Red skin, tiny vesicles on "puffy" surface, scaling, exudation with wet crusts, and cracks (fissures)

DISTRIBUTION   Regional, especially the face (sparing the mouth), the antecubital and popliteal fossae, wrists, and lateral aspects of the legs

CHARACTERISTIC PATTERN   See Figure III.

TREATMENT

Influence of dietary measures at best uncertain. Prompt response to corticosteroids; after improvement, use low-potency corticosteroids or emollients. For recurrence, return for a short period to the stronger corticosteroids. Beware of skin atrophy. With sensible use, no danger of suppression of pituitary adrenal axis. For extra security, monitor growth curve. Tars (ointments, pastes, and gels) also effective. Reassurance of mother. (See Treatment, page 15)

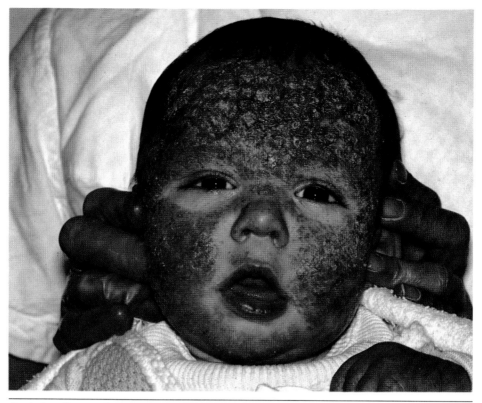

4 Infantile atopic eczema

Patient Profile Five-month-old male infant

History For a month, an itching rash on the face which spread rapidly

Physical Examination On forehead, extensive oozing and crusts on an erythematous skin. Cheeks are diffusely red and erosive; the skin around the eyes and mouth is characteristically normal. Papules on the knees.

Differential Diagnosis Infantile seborrheic eczema

Clues Typical lesions and localization, severe itching. Contrast with seborrheic eczema, which does not itch and has different localization.

Adult-type Atopic Dermatitis

Adult-type atopic dermatitis is a chronic recurrent disease in patients who have or have not had infantile or childhood atopic dermatitis or asthma. Exacerbations are often related to mental stress.

PHYSICAL EXAMINATION

Skin Lesions

TYPE Papular and lichenified plaques, excoriations, pustules, erosions, dry and wet crusts, and cracks (fissures) (see page 371)

DISTRIBUTION Often generalized with predilection for the flexures, front and sides of the neck, eyelids, forehead, face, wrists, and dorsa of feet and hands

TREATMENT

See page 15.

Papaverine hydrochloride 150 mg tid is helpful but has never been proved with controlled studies.

Staphylococcal infection is quite common and, in acute flare-ups, oral antibiotics are indicated, given over a period of weeks.

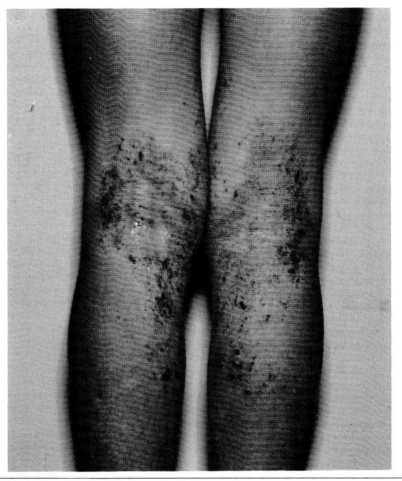

5 Atopic eczematous dermatitis

Patient Profile *Twenty-eight-year-old female typist*

History *For 9 years, a dermatosis was noted, first on the hands; during the past few months the eruption became generalized. There is severe itching. Exacerbations often occur following emotional stress. The skin disease has been a major problem in her social and professional contacts.*

Physical Examination *The lesions involve both popliteal and antecubital fossae, the face, and hands. The lesions include lichenification, erosions, and crusts.*

Differential Diagnosis *Contact dermatitis*

Laboratory and Special Examinations *Patch tests: negative. Bacteriologic culture: a few coagulase-positive* Staphylococcus aureus *sensitive for all tested antibiotics.*

Clues *Clinical picture, severe pruritus, and negative examinations for contact allergy*

Management *Patient was admitted to the hospital for topical corticosteroids and bland topical treatment, without oral antibiotics. Patient was discharged on topical corticosteroids and received guidance from a psychiatrist and psychiatric social worker. Because of their disappointing results, neither scratch nor intradermal tests with so-called atopens are performed any longer in the Leiden Dermatological Department, nor were examinations for IgE or RAST. The positive bacterial culture pointed to colonization, not to infection.*

Childhood-type Atopic Dermatitis

PHYSICAL EXAMINATION

Skin Lesions

TYPE   Papular, lichenified plaques, erosions, crusts

DISTRIBUTION   Especially on the antecubital and popliteal fossae. See Figure III.

TREATMENT

See pages 15 and 18.

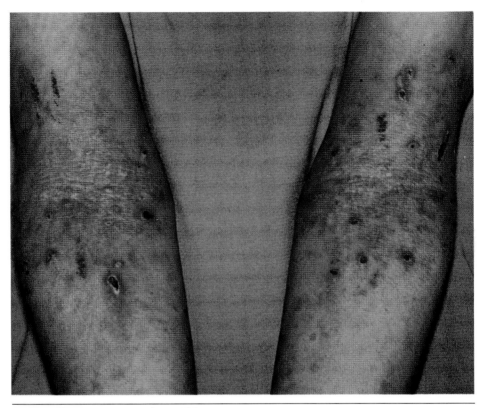

6 Atopic eczematous dermatitis

Patient Profile Eighteen-year-old male

History Since the second year of life, itching dermatosis, and, later, asthma. Frequent secondary infections

Physical Examination In both flexural aspects of the arms, regional lichenifications, erythema, excoriations, and crusts (similar lesions in bends of the knees); also papules and erosions disseminated over the trunk and extremities; pustules on the scalp

Laboratory Examinations Bacterial culture: secondary infection with β-hemolytic group A streptococcus

Clues History, clinical findings (localization to antecubital fossae and lichenification)

Treatment Short course of systemic antibiotics and topical hydrocortisone ointment during hospital treatment

Lichen Simplex (Localized Lichenified Dermatitis)

Lichen simplex is a circumscribed area of lichenification resulting from repeated physical trauma (rubbing and scratching), occurring especially in women on the nuchal areas, arms, legs, and ankles, or in both sexes in the anogenital area.

EPIDEMIOLOGY

Age Over 20 years
Sex More frequent in women
Race A higher incidence in Asians

HISTORY

Duration of Lesion(s) Weeks to months
Skin Symptoms Pruritus, often in paroxysms. The lichenified skin becomes like an erogenous zone—being a pleasure to scratch (orgiastic). Often the areas on the feet are rubbed at night with the heel. The rubbing becomes automatic and reflexive and an unconscious habit.

PHYSICAL EXAMINATION

Skin Lesions

TYPE A solid plaque of lichenification; scaling is minimal except in nuchal lichen simplex.
COLOR Brown or black hyperpigmentation, especially in Skin Types IV, V, and VI (see Appendix D for definitions)
SHAPE Round, oval, linear (following path of scratching)
DISTRIBUTION Isolated single lesion or several scattered plaques (see Figure IV)
CHARACTERISTIC SITES Nuchal area (female), scalp, ankles, lower legs, upper thighs, exterior forearms, vulva, pubis, anal area, scrotum

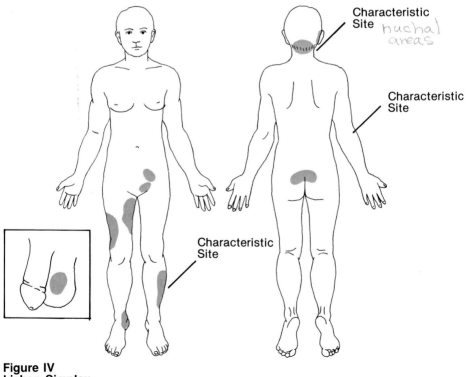

Characteristic Site nuchal areas

Characteristic Site

Characteristic Site

Characteristic Site

Figure IV
Lichen Simplex

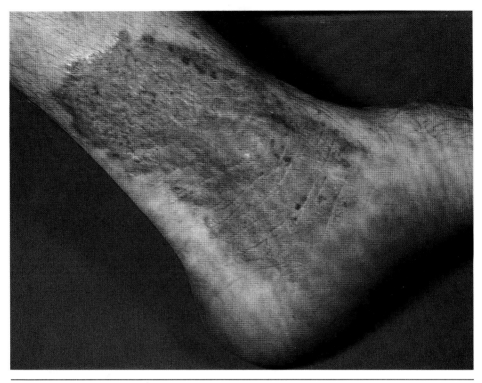

7 Lichen simplex chronicus

Patient Profile *Thirty-four-year-old male*
History *For 2 years, itching patch on medial aspect of right ankle*
Physical Examination *A regional erythematous lichenified plaque with a diameter of 12 cm*
Differential Diagnosis *Lichen planus, lichen amyloidosis*
Clues *Clinical and dermatopathologic aspect, itching*
Treatment *Improvement under treatment with strong topical corticosteroids under plastic occlusion*

DIFFERENTIAL DIAGNOSIS

Lichenification can occur in the absence of atopy, as in psoriasis, mycosis fungoides, or contact dermatitis (chronic) (see page 371).

DERMATOPATHOLOGY

Hyperplasia of all components of epidermis: hyperkeratosis, acanthosis, and elongated and broad rete ridges. Spongiosis is infrequent. In the dermis there is a chronic inflammatory infiltrate.

PATHOPHYSIOLOGY

A special predilection of the skin to respond to physical trauma by epidermal hyperplasia; skin becomes highly sensitive to touch, which is probably related to proliferation of nerves in the epidermis.

TREATMENT

Difficult! The rubbing and scratching must be stopped and hospital treatment is sometimes necessary to completely suppress the scratching with anti-inflammatory agents (topical corticosteroids and crude coal tar) covered by continuous dry occlusive gauze dressings. For small localized areas, intralesional corticosteroids are often highly effective. It is important to apply occlusive bandages at night to prevent rubbing and to facilitate penetration of topical corticosteroids; new occlusive dressings (Actiderm) are very effective.

Nummular (Discoid) Eczema

Discoid eczema is a chronic, pruritic, inflammatory dermatitis occurring in the form of coin-shaped plaques comprised of grouped small papules and vesicles on an erythematous base, especially common on the lower legs of older males during winter months.

EPIDEMIOLOGY

Age and Sex Fifty to eighty years in males; 20 to 40 years in females; infants (as part of atopic dermatitis)

HISTORY

Duration of Lesions Weeks, with remissions and recurrences
Skin Symptoms Pruritus, often intense

PHYSICAL EXAMINATION

Skin Lesions

TYPE

Closely grouped, small vesicles and papules that coalesce into plaques, often more than 4 to 5 cm, with an erythematous base with indistinct borders, crusts, and excoriations
Dry scaly plaques that may be lichenified (see page 371)

COLOR Dull red
SHAPE Round or coin-shaped, hence the adjective nummular (Latin *nummularis*, "like a coin")

DISTRIBUTION

Extent Regional clusters of lesions (e.g., legs) or generalized
Pattern Random
Sites of predilection Lower legs (older men), hands and fingers (younger females)

DIFFERENTIAL DIAGNOSIS

In a single plaque, *dermatophytosis* must be excluded by a potassium hydroxide examination of crusts or scales. *Contact dermatitis* must be excluded by history and localization. *Psoriasis* and *mycosis fungoi-*des may simulate nummular eczema—a biopsy is helpful.

LABORATORY AND SPECIAL EXAMINATIONS

Dermatopathology

SITE Predominantly epidermal
PROCESS Acute inflammation with acanthosis, intraepidermal vesicles, and spongiosis

Microbiologic Examination

DIRECT MICROSCOPIC EXAMINATION OF CRUSTS AND EXUDATE Gram's stain reveals intracellular gram-positive cocci (variable)
CULTURE *Staphylococcus aureus*

PATHOPHYSIOLOGY

A curious variety of the eczematous reaction pattern, often with heavy colonization of staphylococci, frequently occurring in the asteatotic (dry) skin of older men during winter and starting under woolen stockings

COURSE AND PROGNOSIS

Remissions with treatment but frequent recurrences unless the skin is kept hydrated and lubricated

TREATMENT

Oral dicloxacillin or erythromycin
Topical corticosteroids
Crude coal tar pastes with corticosteroids very effective, if tolerated
Hydration of skin with oil water baths followed by application of water-in-oil ointments (hydrated petrolatum)
See Treatment, page 15.

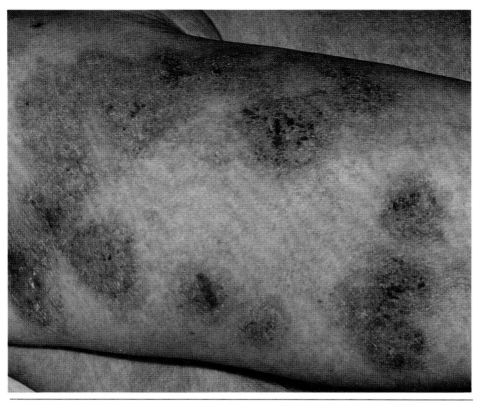

8 Nummular eczematous dermatitis

Patient Profile Sixty-five-year-old female homemaker

History Under treatment for 9 months for rheumatoid arthritis. For 3 weeks, a gradually spreading, itching eruption.

Physical Examination Sharply demarcated, coin-shaped, erythematous, slightly erosive macules disseminated diffusely over trunk, upper arms, and thighs

Differential Diagnosis Drug eruption

Laboratory and Special Examinations Fungi and bacteria: negative.

Clues Typical coin-shaped eczematous lesions

Pompholyx (A Special Vesicular Type of Hand and Foot Eczema)

Pompholyx is an acute, chronic or recurrent dermatosis of the fingers, palms, and soles characterized by a sudden onset of deep-seated pruritic, clear, "sago-like" vesicles; later, scaling, fissures, lichenification occur. Secondary bacterial infection is very often a complication.

EPIDEMIOLOGY

Age Majority under 40 years (range 12–40 years)
Sex Equal ratio

HISTORY

Duration of Lesions Onset in a few days
Skin Symptoms Pruritus and especially painful fissures that are incapacitating. Summer exacerbations are not infrequent.

PHYSICAL EXAMINATION

Skin Lesions

TYPE

Early Vesicles, usually small (1.0 mm), deep-seated, appearing like "tapioca" in clusters, occasionally bullae, especially on the feet
Later Scaling, lichenification, painful fissures, and erosions
ARRANGEMENT Vesicles grouped in clusters
DISTRIBUTION Regional [hands (80%) and feet] with sites of predilection bilaterally on the sides of fingers, palms, and soles
NAILS Dystrophic changes (transverse ridging, pitting, and thickening)
Hyperhidrosis is present in some patients

DIFFERENTIAL DIAGNOSIS

Vesicular reaction to active dermatophytosis on the feet; acute contact dermatitis.

DERMATOPATHOLOGY

Site Epidermis
Process Eczematous inflammation (spongiosis and intraepidermal edema) with subcorneal vesicles usually unrelated to sweat ducts

PATHOPHYSIOLOGY

Despite the name sometimes used, dyshidrotic eczema, there is little evidence that sweating plays a role in the pathogenesis.

About half the patients have an atopic background. Emotional stress is possibly a precipitating factor. The role of nickel ingestion in the diet is unsettled. Lesions can be induced by ingestion of high doses of nickel. Hyperhidrosis may or may not be present. The term pompholyx (Greek, "bubble") is preferred until the pathogenesis is settled.

COURSE AND PROGNOSIS

Recurrent attacks with intervals of weeks to months with spontaneous remissions in 2 to 3 weeks.

TREATMENT

A frustrating experience. Avoid systemic corticosteroids except in rare, short-term flare-ups; patients can become dependent on low-dose corticosteroids and serious complications can occur.

Vesicular stage (early) Burow's wet dressings; large bullae should be drained but not unroofed. Small vesicles respond dramatically but unpredictably to "black cat" applied once daily. Black cat is 10% crude coal tar in equal parts of acetone and flexible collodion.

Eczematous stage (later) With fissures, scaling, lichenification. Topical corticosteroids are unpredictably successful in a few patients but should be tried. High-potency corticosteroids (e.g., clobetasol-17-proprionate) should be tried with proper warning about cutaneous and systemic side effects.

Bacterial infection may be present even without obvious signs (crusts, tenderness, etc.) and erythromycin 250 mg qid should be started in most patients with moderate or severe disease.

Diet restriction of certain metals (nickel, cobalt, or chromium) has been suggested to be successful in two-thirds of the patients in one series.

PUVA (oral or topical as "soaks") is successful in a few patients and is worth trying, especially in severe pompholyx.

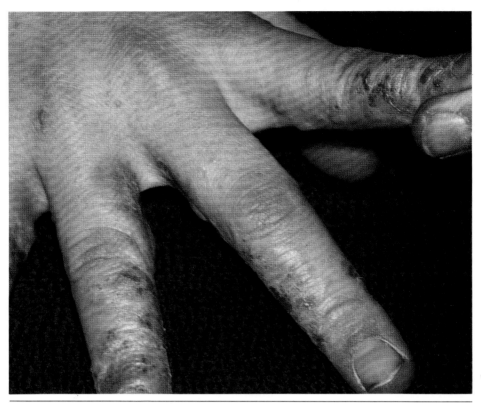

9 Dyshidrotic eczematous dermatitis

Patient Profile Twelve-year-old male

History For 14 days, an itching eruption of the hands

Physical Examination Itching vesicles, a few pustules and erosions disseminated over dorsa and interdigital spaces of fingers

Differential Diagnosis Contact eczematous dermatitis, eczematous dermatophytosis

Laboratory and Special Examinations Mycologic examination: negative.

Clues Negative examinations for fungi, bacteria, and allergens. No history of contact dermatitis.

Course and Prognosis In spite of treatment with corticosteroid cream, spreading occurred, with large bullae on the palms, papules disseminated over the trunk, and papulovesicular eruptions on the legs and feet, necessitating hospital admission. Bacterial culture negative.

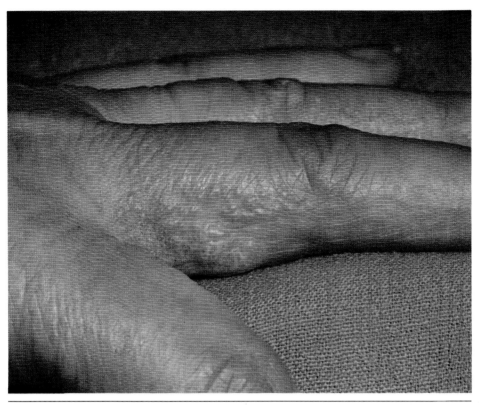

10 Dyshidrotic eczematous dermatitis

Patient Profile Forty-seven-year-old female homemaker

History For 14 years, a rash on the hands with remissions and exacerbations

Physical Examination Deep-seated vesicles of firm consistency appearing "like tapioca" along the sides of the fingers. No lesions between toes or on the feet.

Differential Diagnosis Dermatophytid, eczematous contact dermatitis.

Laboratory Examinations Mycologic examination of vesicle roof and scales of the feet: negative. Patch tests with a standard screening tray: negative.

Stasis dermatitis is a recalcitrant chronic dermatitis of the lower legs in persons with chronic venous insufficiency; ulceration occurs frequently.

EPIDEMIOLOGY

Age Over 50 years
Sex More common in women

HISTORY

Duration of Lesions Months
Skin Symptoms Mild pruritus, pain (if ulcer present)
Other Features Aching discomfort in the limb, swelling of the ankle, nocturnal cramps

PHYSICAL EXAMINATION

Skin Lesions

TYPE

Erythematous scaling plaque with exudation, crusts, and superficial ulcers (see Figure 11)
Brown reticulated hemosiderin hyperpigmentation (on ankles and lower legs)

SHAPE Round or oval

DISTRIBUTION

Extent Localized
Sites of predilection Medial aspect of ankle (Figure 11)

DIFFERENTIAL DIAGNOSIS

Primary varicose veins are hereditary, often unilateral. The *postphlebitic limb* is associated with the most severe venous stasis and the ulcers are usually larger. Fibrosing panniculitis with firm tender induration may be observed.

In the absence of the typical pigmentation and small-vein enlargement of venous stasis, the diagnosis of stasis dermatitis is suspect and other causes for ulcers should be considered, such as *organic disease of arteries, carcinoma, cryoglobulinemia, sickle cell anemia, necrobiosis lipoidica, pyoderma gangrenosum.*

TREATMENT

Stasis Dermatitis

ACUTE Burow's wet dressings and cooling pastes and later topical corticosteroids; systemic antibiotics if cellulitis is present
CHRONIC Elevation of the leg
Ulcer
Wet to dry dressings. Silver sulfadiazine (Silvadene) applied between wet to dry dressings. Zinc gelatin bandage, elevation of the leg, supportive stockings. For larger persistent ulcers, daily applications of allografts (cadaver skin) are very effective. Supportive stockings and surgery are necessary adjuncts to topical therapy.

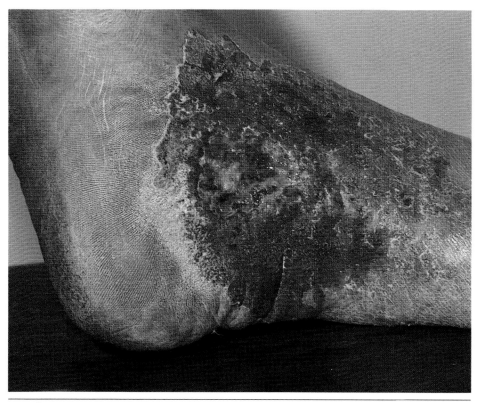

11 Stasis dermatitis and ulcer

Patient Profile Fifty-two-year-old female homemaker

History For 5 years, painful ulcers on the right ankle, no preceding venous thrombosis.

Physical Examination Multiple, grouped, irregularly demarcated, shallow ulcerations with yellow base, surrounded by an erythematous oozing area. Venous stasis and edema

Differential Diagnosis Infectious eczematous dermatitis, contact eczematous dermatitis

Laboratory Examinations Venous stasis and edema. Bacteriologic culture: Pseudomonas aeruginosa

Clues Edema, clinical picture, negative patch tests

Treatment Treatment of venous stasis with compressive bandages, combined with wet dressings with silver nitrate alternated with cooling pastes. Maintenance treatment of stasis with supportive stockings.

Diaper Dermatitis

Diaper dermatitis is an acute inflammatory dermatosis resulting from prolonged exposure to urine or feces or irritant chemicals in the diaper.

EPIDEMIOLOGY

Age Onset after first 6 weeks and highest occurrence up to 5 months. May occur in incontinent older persons.

HISTORY

Duration of Lesions Weeks
Skin Symptoms Pruritus, burning, pain

PHYSICAL EXAMINATION

Skin Lesions

TYPE Erythema (like a heat burn), vesicles, erosions–ulcers, papules
COLOR Bright red

DISTRIBUTION

Extent Regional, where diaper covers skin, but can involve upper thighs and lower abdomen
Pattern Body folds usually spared. See Figure 12.

DIFFERENTIAL DIAGNOSIS

Intertrigo (erythema only); *candidiasis* (sharp margins, raised scaling edges); *seborrheic dermatitis* (yellow greasy scales and scalp involvement); *miliaria* (papules and vesicles)

PATHOPHYSIOLOGY

Chemical burn from ammonia produced by the bacterial decomposition of urea. Factors that favor development: infrequent diaper changes, diarrhea, humid hot ambient temperature, occlusive plastic pants. Harsh chemicals in the diaper itself may be a contributing cause.

TREATMENT

Frequent diaper change with bathing of area covered by the diaper, copious use of "baby" powder
Topical low-potency corticosteroids in ointment bases used for short periods only
Application of zinc oxide paste to prevent recurrences
Avoid plastic occlusive pants
Air dry (eliminate diapers for a few hours)

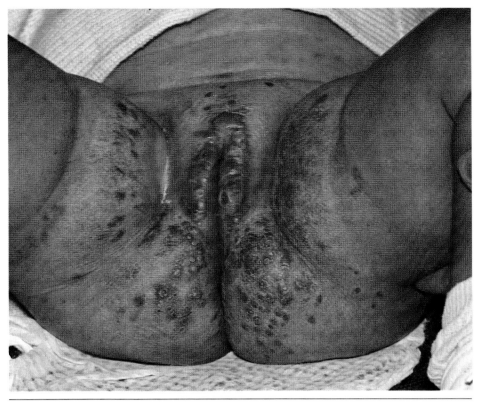

12 Diaper dermatitis

Patient Profile Six-month-old female infant

History For 2 months, a rash involving vulva, buttocks, inguinal folds

Physical Examination Vulva, buttocks, and thighs diffusely red. On buttocks, disseminated flat papules with some erosions (white color due to zinc oxide ointment).

Differential Diagnosis Seborrheic dermatitis, intertriginous candidiasis, diaper dermatitis

Laboratory Examination Examination for Candida: negative.

Clues Negative mycologic examination, localization, presence of circumscribed erosions; less diffuse than seborrheic dermatitis

Treatment Bland pastes (e.g., zinc oxide), frequent changes of diaper, avoidance of plastic pants

Asteatotic Dermatitis (Eczema Craquelé[1])

Asteatotic dermatitis is a relatively common dermatitis that occurs in the winter and in older persons on the legs, arms, and hands and is characterized by dry, "cracked," fissured skin.

EPIDEMIOLOGY

Age Over 40 years
Sex More common in males

HISTORY

Duration of Lesions Weeks, months
Skin Symptoms Pruritus
Other Factors Often a history of over-bathing

PHYSICAL EXAMINATION

Skin Lesions

TYPE Dry "cracked" skin (see Figures 13 and 14) with red fissures and slight scaling, and sometimes lichenification [see Discoid (Nummular) Eczema]
ARRANGEMENT Diffuse skin involvement (without identifiable borders), irregular reticulation

DISTRIBUTION

Extent Generalized
Sites of predilection Legs, dorsa of hands and forearms

DERMATOPATHOLOGY

Site Epidermis
Process Eczema with spongiosis and mild dermal infiltrate

PATHOPHYSIOLOGY

Asteatosis (loss of lipids) can occur with overbathing, old age, a genetic tendency for dry skin (not necessarily ichthyosis), and high environmental temperature with low relative humidity (as in heated rooms).

TREATMENT

Increase ambient humidity, preferably above 50 percent
Tepid water baths containing bath oils with immediate liberal application of emollient ointments
Wool should be substituted by cotton
Room humidifiers (in the bedroom) are very helpful

---

[1] The term *craquelé* is a French word meaning "marred with cracks," as in old china or ceramic tile.

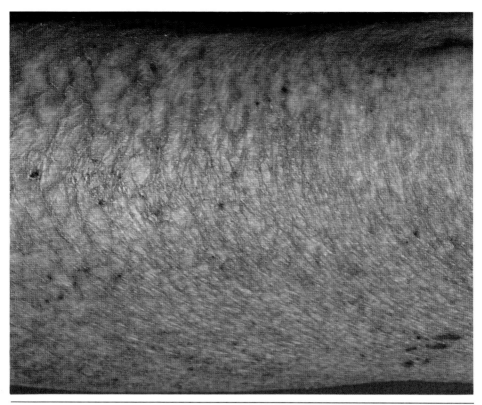

13 Eczema craquelé
Asteatotic eczema

Patient Profile Sixty-nine-year-old male

History Gradually extending eruption over the whole body in a patient with an inoperable stomach cancer. Referred with a question of drug eruption due to barbiturates.

Physical Examination Diffuse network of chapping over the skin, transforming partially into red fissures with scaling border

Differential Diagnosis Drug eruption

Clues Typical lesions

Pathophysiology The chapping and subsequent changes are due to water loss in the stratum corneum.

Treatment A reduction of soap bathing and the addition of water-oil baths followed by the application of an emollient, which diminishes water loss from the stratum corneum, resulted in rapid improvement.

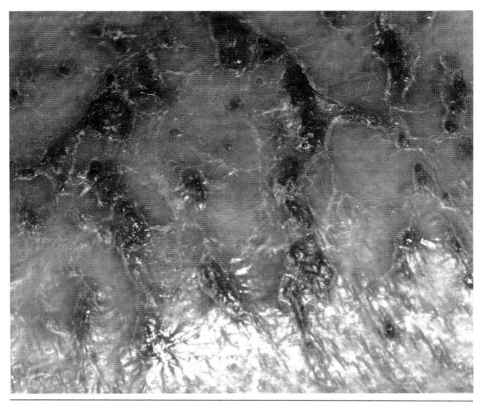

14 Eczema craquelé
   Asteatotic eczema

Detail of Figure 13

II
Drug Eruptions

Drug Eruptions Due to Hypersensitivity Mechanisms

Drug eruptions can mimic virtually all the morphologic expressions in dermatology and must be first on the differential diagnosis in the appearance of a sudden symmetrical eruption. The majority are based on a hypersensitivity mechanism: types I, II, III, and IV.

Drug eruptions are caused by immunologic or nonimmunologic mechanisms and are provoked by systemic or topical administration of a drug. The immunologic drug reactions may be of types I, II, III, or IV. The nonimmunologic drug eruptions are caused by (1) idiosyncrasy *sensu strictirori*—reactions due to hereditary enzyme deficiencies; (2) cumulation, such as melanosis due to gold or Cordarone; (3) irritancy of a topically applied drug; (4) an individual hypersensitivity to a topical or systemic drug; (5) mechanisms not yet known; and (6) reactions due to the combination of a drug with ultraviolet irradiation (photosensitivity). These may have a toxic (T) or immunologic (allergic) (A) pathology.

Photosensitivity after systemic administration:

Phenothiazines	A + T
Chlorpromazine (Largactil)	
Promethazine (Phenergan)	
Sulfanilamides	A + T
Oral antidiabetics	
Sulfanilureum derivatives	
Demethylchlortetracycline (Declomycin)	T
Other tetracyclines more rarely	
Nalidixic acid	T
Amino hydrochloride (Cordarone)	T

Photosensitivity after topical application:

Pix lithantracis	T
Phenothiazines	A + T
Sulfonamides	A + T
A number of halogenated salicylanilides	A
Bithionol	A

EPIDEMIOLOGY AND ETIOLOGY

Age Occur at any age
Sex More common in females
Incidence The most common manifestation of drug sensitivity; affect 3.0 percent of hospitalized patients in the United States—about half are minor and less than 10 percent are serious

Most Frequent Types

EXANTHEMATOUS Penicillin, ampicillin, barbiturates, phenylbutazone, gold, quinidine, sulfonamides, allopurinol, phenytoin
URTICARIA Penicillins, salicylates, erythromycin (see page 118)
PHOTOSENSITIVITY Sulfonamide diuretics and antidiabetics, phenothiazines, nalidixic acid, tetracycline, Declomycin, vinblastin, nonsteroidal anti-inflammatory agents
FIXED DRUG (See Figure 16) Phenolphthalein, barbiturates, phenacetin, sulfonamides, tetracycline
PURPURA (NONTHROMBOCYTOPENIC) Thiazides, carbromal (see Figure 15), type II (cytotoxic) reactions
BULLOUS Barbiturates, iodides, sulfonamides, penicillin
SERUM SICKNESS Penicillin, salicylates, sulfonamides, barbiturates
ERYTHEMA MULTIFORME SYNDROME Sulfonamides, phenytoin, barbiturates, phenylbutazone, penicillin (see page 122)
OTHER LESS FREQUENT TYPES Acneform, toxic epidermal necrolysis, necrotizing vasculitis, erythema nodosum

HISTORY

Duration of Lesions Usually appear within first week except reactions due to ampicillin and other semisynthetic penicillins, when eruptions may be delayed
Skin Symptoms Pruritus—mild, severe, or absent

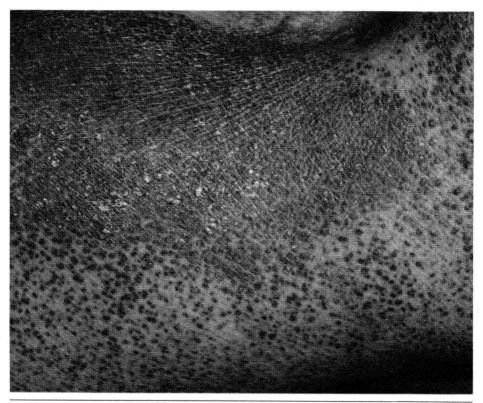

15 Drug eruption (carbromal)

Patient Profile Fifty-eight-year-old male

History For 7 days, a rash over trunk and lower legs

Physical Examination Moderately itching eruption of brown-red, pinpoint to larger macules and papules scattered discretely and in places confluent. Some lichenified, slightly scaling patches. Patient is a poor sleeper and takes sleeping tablets.

Differential Diagnosis Schamberg's progressive pigmentary disease

Clues History and typical clinical aspect

Treatment Discontinuation of carbromal

PHYSICAL EXAMINATION

Skin Lesions

TYPE

    Maculopapular (morbilliform or scarlatiniform)
    Urticarial wheal
    Vesicular and bullous
    Purpuric macules or papules (vasculitis)

COLOR

Exanthematous eruptions Bright "drug red"
Fixed-drug eruptions Dusky red or violaceous
SHAPE Round, oval, polycyclic, annular, iris
ARRANGEMENT Scattered discrete lesions

DISTRIBUTION

    Isolated single lesion (fixed-drug)
    Generalized

SITES OF PREDILECTION

Fixed drug Legs, hands, glans penis
Exanthematous Trunk, may be generalized

Urticaria Generalized, hands and feet, lips, eyelids

DIAGNOSIS

Detailed history with list of all medications taken by mouth, by injection, and proprietary preparations for headache, sleep, cold, constipation, pain, etc.

No laboratory tests are available at present that can establish the diagnosis; RAST correlates well with skin-test reactivity in penicillin-sensitive patients.

COURSE

Progression may continue for a while, but in most cases the eruption disappears within days after the offending drug is stopped.

TREATMENT

Systemic corticosteroids are frequently used for severe reactions, although their efficacy has not been proved.

Antihistamines are helpful in some urticarial drug eruptions.

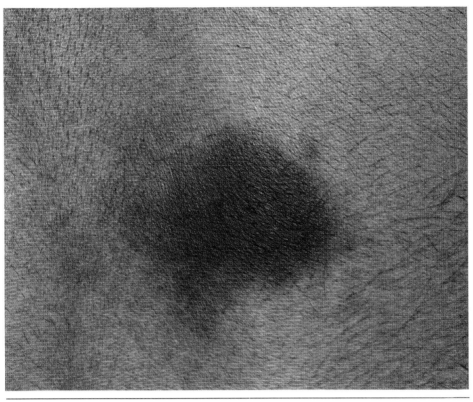

16 Fixed-drug eruption

Patient Profile Forty-three-year-old female

History For 5 months, at irregular intervals, at the same site on the leg violet spots arise, which disappear after some time. Patient is taking, at irregular intervals, a phenazone-containing analgesic.

Physical Examination A violet, irregularly bordered plaque

Differential Diagnosis Purpura

Clues Clinical morphology and history

Treatment Discontinuation of phenazone

III
The Psoriasis
Syndromes

The Psoriasis Syndromes

Psoriasis, which affects 1.5 to 2.0 percent of the population in western countries, is an hereditary disorder of skin with several clinical expressions—but most typically chronic scaling papules and plaques in a characteristic distribution, largely at sites of repeated minor trauma.

EPIDEMIOLOGY AND ETIOLOGY

Age One-third of patients before 20 years of age, especially in females

Sex Equal in males and females

Race Low incidence in West Africans, American Indians, and Japanese

Other Features Multifactorial inheritance. Minor trauma (Koebner's phenomenon) is a major factor (45 percent of patients) in eliciting lesions. Certain drugs (systemic corticosteroids, lithium, alcohol, chloroquine), sunlight, stress, and obesity are believed to cause exacerbation of preexisting psoriasis.

HISTORY

Duration of Lesions Usually months but may be sudden as in acute guttate psoriasis and generalized pustular psoriasis (von Zumbusch)

Skin Symptoms Pruritus is reasonably common, especially in scalp and anogenital psoriasis

Constitutional Symptoms Arthritis, fever, and "acute illness" syndrome (weakness, chills, fever) with generalized pustular psoriasis (von Zumbusch)

PHYSICAL EXAMINATION

Skin Lesions

TYPE

Papules and plaques with marked silvery-white scaling, sharply marginated (see Figures 17 to 20 and 22)
Pustules (see Figures 23 and 24)
Erythroderma

COLOR "Salmon pink"

SHAPE Round, oval, polycyclic, annular

ARRANGEMENT Zosteriform, arciform, serpiginous, scattered discrete lesions, or erythroderma (diffuse involvement without identifiable borders)

DISTRIBUTION

Extent Single lesion or lesions localized to one area (e.g., penis), regional involvement (scalp), generalized or universal (entire skin, nails)

Pattern (1) Bilateral, rarely symmetrical, spares exposed areas, favors sites of pressure and intertriginous areas. For characteristic pattern of distribution, see Figure V. (2) Disseminated small lesions ("guttate" psoriasis) see page 51 and Figure 18).

Hair and Nails

Hair loss (alopecia) is not a common feature even with severe scalp involvement.

Fingernails (see Figure 21) and toenails frequently (25 percent) involved, especially with concomitant arthritis. Nail changes include: pitting (Figure 21) (frequent but nonspecific), onycholysis (also nonspecific), and yellow spots under the nail plate—the "oil spot" (pathognomonic!).

Arthritis

Incidence is uncertain (1 to 32 percent). Incidence of seronegative psoriatic arthritis in hospitalized patients is 7 percent.
Rare before age 20.
Two types: (1) "distal"—seronegative and without subcutaneous nodules, involving terminal interphalangeal joints of hands and feet; (2) mutilating psoriatic arthritis with bone erosion and osteolysis and, ultimately, ankylosis; especially involving the sacroiliac, hip, and cervical areas with ankylosing spondylitis; seen especially in erythrodermic and pustular psoriasis.

DIFFERENTIAL DIAGNOSIS

Seborrheic dermatitis—may be indistinguishable in sites involved and morphology; *lichen simplex chronicus*—may complicate psoriasis due to pruritus; *candidiasis*—especially confused with intertriginous psoriasis; *psoriasiform drug eruptions*—especially beta blockers, gold, and methyldopa; *glucagonoma syndrome*—important differential as this is a serious disease (malignant tumor of pan-

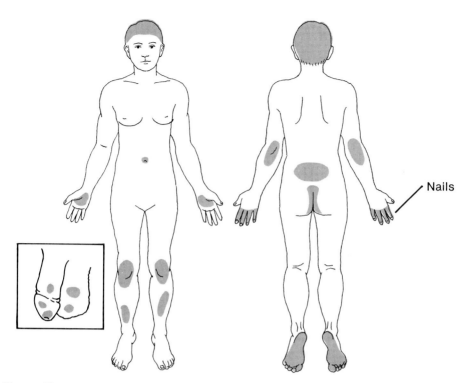

Figure V
Psoriasis

creatic islet cells). The psoriasiform lesions are atypical—annular lesions but with vesicles and erosions. Distinguishing features include lesions in groin and on face, marked weight loss, unexplained anemia, intermittent diarrhea, stomatitis; the histology is quite specific.

DERMATOPATHOLOGY

Site Epidermis and dermis

Process Inflammation plus alteration of the cell cycle. There is (1) marked thickening and also thinning of the epidermis with elongation of the rete ridges; (2) increased mitosis of keratinocytes, fibroblasts, and endothelial cells; (3) parakeratotic hyperkeratosis (nuclei retained in the stratum corneum); and (4) inflammatory cells in the dermis (usually lymphocytes and monocytes) and in the epidermis (polymorphonuclear cells), forming microabscesses of Munro in the stratum corneum.

PATHOPHYSIOLOGY

Psoriasis probably refers to a cluster of diseases of differing pathogenesis. The principal abnormality in psoriasis is an alteration of the cell kinetics of keratino-cytes. The major change is a shortening of the cell cycle from 311 to 36 hours; this results in production of 35,000 cells per day, 28 times the normal production, 1246 cells per day. The etiologic basis for this increased production is not known. The epidermis and dermis appear to respond as an integrated system: the primary changes in the keratogenous zone of the epidermis and the inflammatory changes in the dermis, which may "trigger" the epidermal changes. The level of cyclic nucleotides is altered (decreased cyclic AMP), but it is not known whether this is a primary or secondary control mechanism for keratinocyte proliferation.

TREATMENT

It is difficult to generalize regarding treatment of psoriasis as the selection of the several therapies depends on (1) the type of psoriasis, (2) stage of the disease (acute or chronic), (3) the site (e.g., scalp vs. intertriginous), (4) the extent of the disease, (5) the age of the patient, and (6) the degree of disability or disfigurement.

The major categories are illustrated in Figures 17 to 24, and the treatment is presented.

Localized Plaques of Psoriasis

TREATMENT

Instruct the patient that he or she should never rub or scratch the lesions as this trauma stimulates the psoriatic proliferative process (Koebner's phenomenon).

Treatment only with topically administered agents.

1. Topical fluorinated corticosteroids (betamethasone valerate, fluocinolone acetonide, betamethasone propionate) in ointment base applied after removing the scales by soaking in water. The ointment is applied to the wet skin, covered with plastic wrap, and left on overnight.

2. Use of Actiderm (left on for 24–48 hours) is helpful and effective and prevents scratching. During the day fluorinated corticosteroid creams can be used without occlusion. Patients will develop tolerance after long periods. Caveat: Prolonged application of the fluorinated corticosteroids leads to atrophy of the skin and unsightly telangiectasia. Clobetasol-17-propionate is stronger and active even without occlusion. To avoid systemic effects: maximum 50 g ointment a week.

3. For very small plaques (4.0 cm or less) triamcinolone acetonide, aqueous suspension, 5.0 mg/ml is injected into the lesion 0.1 ml/mm^2. The injection should be intradermal rather than subcutaneous; if the injection does not require some pressure to inject, *it is not going into the dermis. Warning:* Atrophic macules can result.

4. Topical anthralin preparations are excellent when used properly. Follow directions on the package insert with attention to details.

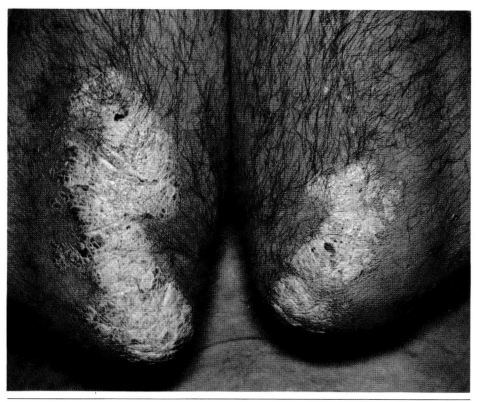

17 Psoriasis vulgaris

Patient Profile Fifty-five-year-old male

History For 25 years, generalized nonpruritic red patches covered with thick white scales. Flares are often associated with nervous stress. Father and one uncle have similar lesions.

Physical Examination On the extensor surface of the elbows, erythematous patches covered with silvery-white keratotic plaques. Similar lesions on extensor surfaces of knees, lower legs, and scalp.

Differential Diagnosis Seborrheic dermatitis, psoriasiform drug eruption from beta blockers

Clues Circumscribed white-scaling plaques, sites of predilection

Psoriasis Vulgaris, Guttate Type

This type of psoriasis, which is relatively rare (less than 2.0 percent of all psoriasis), is like an exanthem: a shower of lesions appearing rather rapidly in young adults and often following streptococcal pharyngitis. Guttate psoriasis may, however, be chronic and unrelated to streptococcal infection.

PHYSICAL EXAMINATION

Skin Lesions

TYPE Papules 2.0 mm to 1.0 cm
COLOR "Salmon pink"
SHAPE Guttate (Latin, "spots that resemble drops")
ARRANGEMENT Scattered discrete lesions
DISTRIBUTION Generalized, usually sparing the palms and soles and concentrating on the trunk, less on the face, scalp, and nails

DIFFERENTIAL DIAGNOSIS

Psoriasiform drug eruption

LABORATORY EXAMINATION

Serologic: an increased antistreptolysin titer in those patients with antecedent streptococcal infection

COURSE AND PROGNOSIS

Often, but not always, this type of psoriasis spontaneously disappears in a few weeks without treatment.

TREATMENT

The resolution of lesions can be accelerated by UVB phototherapy or judicious exposure to sunlight. For persistent lesions, treatment same as for generalized plaque psoriasis (see page 54).

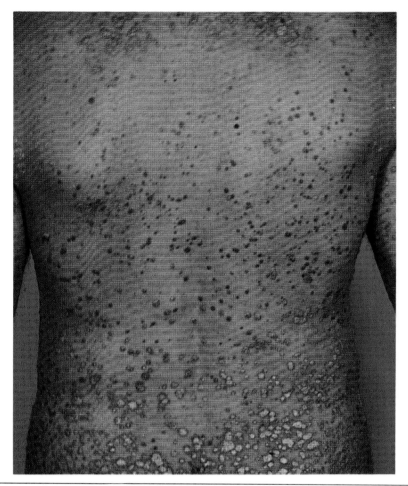

18 Psoriasis guttata (guttate psoriasis)

Patient Profile Thirty-four-year-old female

History For 15 years, nonpruritic rash on the trunk and extremities. Variable course, exacerbations probably associated with emotional stress. Improves with sunbathing. Family history noncontributory.

Physical Examination Disseminated over the back are numerous 3- to 10-mm, sharply marginated, slightly indurated patches. Covered in the upper and lower areas with white keratotic scales.

Differential Diagnosis Secondary syphilis, pityriasis rosea

Laboratory and Special Examinations Serologic tests for syphilis: negative. Antistreptolysin titer: normal. Histology: see page 47.

Clues Disseminated red-scaling patches

Treatment Satisfactory response to PUVA maintenance: one treatment every three weeks.

Psoriasis of the Scalp

Psoriasis of the scalp presents a special therapeutic problem, similar to that of anogenital psoriasis. Both areas are inaccessible for phototherapy and are usually pruritic, which results in lichenification and koebnerization.* Psoriasis of the scalp may be part of generalized plaque psoriasis, may coexist with isolated plaques, or may be the only site involved.

HISTORY

Duration   Months to years

Relationship to Season   Does not go into remission with sunlight exposure as does the exposed skin

Skin Symptoms   Mild to severe pruritus, which often causes compulsive and subconscious scratching

PHYSICAL EXAMINATION

Type

Plaques, often with thick adherent scales

Lichenification (often superimposed on the basic psoriatic lesions and resulting from rubbing and scratching)

Exudation and fissures, especially behind the ears

Arrangement   Scattered discrete plaques or diffuse involvement of the entire scalp

(N.B.: Paradoxically, alopecia is an uncommon complication of psoriasis of the scalp, even after years of thick, plaque-type involvement. Thus the condition is not exposed to public view—and may be one reason why patients learn to live with it and do not seek treatment.)

DIFFERENTIAL DIAGNOSIS

Seborrheic dermatitis of the scalp may be almost indistinguishable from psoriasis. Some have called this "seborrhiasis."

PATHOPHYSIOLOGY

There may be a subset of psoriasis of the scalp that could be related to the colonization of pityrosporal yeasts inasmuch as one controlled study showed a beneficial effect of oral and topical ketoconazole.

TREATMENT

Mild (superficial scaling and without thick plaques):
- Tar shampoos followed by
- Betamethasone valerate 0.1% lotion 2 times weekly

Severe (thick adherent plaques):
- Removal of plaques before active treatment. Topical applications are virtually useless unless the thick scale is removed. This is accomplished by applications of 2% salicylic acid in mineral oil, covered with a plastic cap, and left on overnight.
- After scales have been removed (in 1 to 3 treatments), fluocinolone cream is applied and the scalp is covered with plastic sheets or a shower cap, which is left on overnight.
- When the thickness of the plaques is reduced, betamethasone valerate lotion 0.1% can be used for maintenance. *Compulsive subconscious scratching and rubbing will negate all attempts for maintenance treatment. Hands off!*

COURSE AND PROGNOSIS

The prognosis for control is good; following treatment as outlined above, the scalp lesions may undergo a remission for several months to years. Scratching and rubbing must be avoided in order to maintain the remission.

---

*The phenomenon of induction of new lesions on "normal" skin by physical trauma, including rubbing and scratching.

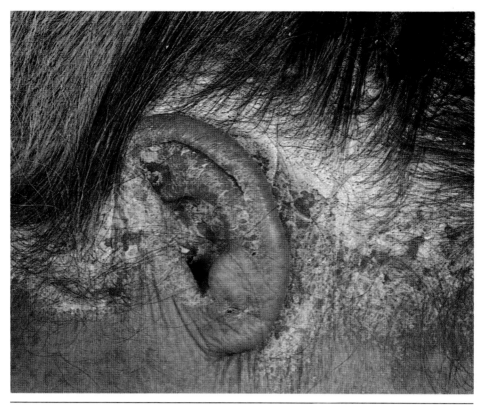

19 Psoriasis of the scalp

Patient Profile Fifty-eight-year-old female

History For 30 years, widespread psoriasis on the scalp, extremities, and trunk. For 5 years, mild arthritis of finger joints.

Physical Examination Thick, silver-white, heavily scaling lesions of the scalp and ear. No hair loss.

Differential Diagnosis Seborrheic dermatitis

Clues Thick silver-white scaling in site of predilection

Treatment Much improved under 0.1% triamcinolone acetonide and 5% salicylic acid in O/W cream with plastic occlusion at night. Later, maintenance with a corticosteroid scalp lotion.

Psoriasis Vulgaris, Generalized Plaque Type

Psoriasis vulgaris is a challenge for the physician, as chronic generalized psoriasis is one of the "miseries that beset mankind," causing shame and embarrassment and a compromised life-style. The "heartbreak of psoriasis" is no joke. As the writer John Updike so poignantly said about a person with psoriasis, "Lusty, though we are loathsome to love. Keen-sighted, though we hate to look upon ourselves. The name of the disease, spiritually speaking, is Humiliation."

TREATMENT

The management of generalized plaque-type psoriasis is the province of a well-qualified dermatologist or of a psoriasis center where there are available the major options: (1) UVB phototherapy with emollients, (2) PUVA photochemotherapy, (3) methotrexate (given weekly), or (4) combination therapy using etretinate or methotrexate with PUVA is perhaps the ideal treatment available at the present time. In our psoriasis population 60 percent respond well to UVB plus emollients when given according to a published protocol. Those who do not respond are treated with oral PUVA photochemotherapy. Methotrexate is used only if UVB or PUVA treatment fails. Etretinate is not used in females nor as a monotherapy. For males, combination etretinate and oral PUVA photochemotherapy is a very effective therapy.

Treatment consists of oral ingestion of 8-methoxypsoralen (8-MOP) (0.3 to 0.6 mg 8-MOP per kg body weight) and exposure to varying doses of UVA depending on the sensitivity of the patient. Approximately 1 h after ingestion of the psoralen, UVA is given starting at a dose of 1 J/cm^2, adjusted upward for skin phototype. The UVA dose is increased by 0.5 to 1.0 J/cm^2 each dose. Treatments are performed 2 or 3 times a week or, if employing a more intensive protocol, 4 times a week. The majority of patients clear after 19 to 25 treatments, and the amount of UVA needed ranges from 100 to 245 J/cm^2. In patients with recalcitrant, plaque-type psoriasis, etretinate may be combined with other antipsoriatic therapy, e.g., PUVA, UVB, topical corticosteroids, anthralin, or methotrexate. These combination modalities have been shown to reduce the length of treatment as well as the total amount of an antipsoriatic drug necessary for clearing. Topical corticosteroids, anthralin, methotrexate, and etretinate, combined with either PUVA or UVB, have all been shown to be effective in reducing the dose of one another.

Psoriasis day-care centers or inpatient services also have available the dithranol technique or UVB plus tar application (Goeckermann regimen) given by a trained staff.

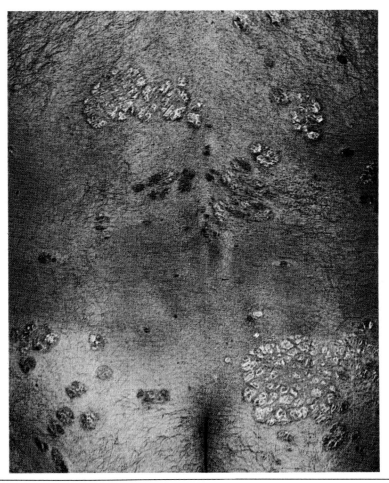

20 Psoriasis vulgaris

Patient Profile *Thirty-one-year-old male*

History *For 6 years, disseminated nonpruritic scaling patches on trunk and extremities*

Physical Examination *On the back, several erythematous patches, 3 to 15 cm in size, slightly indurated, sharply marginated, and with slight scaling, most pronounced peripherally*

Differential Diagnosis *Tinea corporis*

Laboratory and Special Examinations *Histology: see page 47.*

Clues *Sharp demarcation, prolonged duration*

Psoriasis of the Nails

Psoriasis of the nails is quite common (25 percent of patients with psoriasis), varies in severity of involvement, and often disappears spontaneously or with treatment of psoriasis of the skin, especially with the three major treatments: UVB phototherapy, PUVA photochemotherapy, and methotrexate.

TREATMENT

Specially directed treatment of the fingernails (inasmuch as they are disfiguring and a nuisance) is unsatisfactory. Injection of the nail fold with intradermal triamcinolone acetonide (5 mg/ml) is quite effective but almost invariably produces atrophy.

PUVA photochemotherapy is somewhat effective; the ultraviolet A is administered in special hand and foot lighting units providing high-intensity UVA.

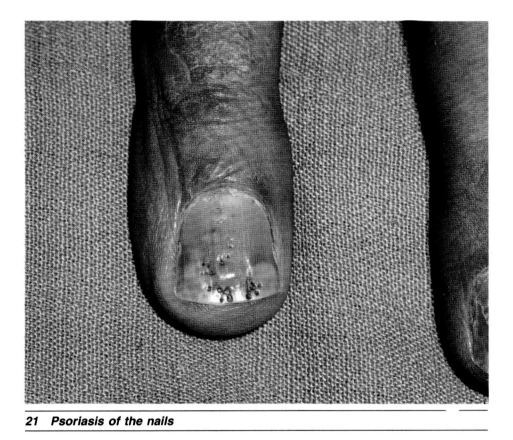

21 Psoriasis of the nails

Same patient as in Figure 20. The nails show distal onycholysis (white-yellowish areas) and discrete punctate pits in the surface ("thimble nails"). On the proximal part of the finger is a delicate psoriasis patch.

Differential Diagnosis Nail changes due to fungal infection or associated with chronic eczema or alopecia areata

Psoriasis Vulgaris of the Palms and Soles

This disease is a major therapeutic challenge. The palms and soles may be the only areas involved. Topical corticosteroids with plastic occlusion are quite ineffective. UVB phototherapy is not often effective. Intralesional triamcinolone acetonide is hazardous because of risks of bacterial infection in the maze of tendons.

TREATMENT

Two quite effective treatments available are

1. PUVA photochemotherapy, administered in specially designed hand and foot lighting cabinets that deliver UVA. UVB phototherapy is not effective for palm and sole involvement of psoriasis.

2. Retinoids (etretinate) given alone orally are sometimes effective in clearing psoriasis vulgaris of the palms and soles. Combinations of oral retinoids and PUVA appear to improve the efficacy of each, and to permit a reduction of the dose and duration of each (see page 54).

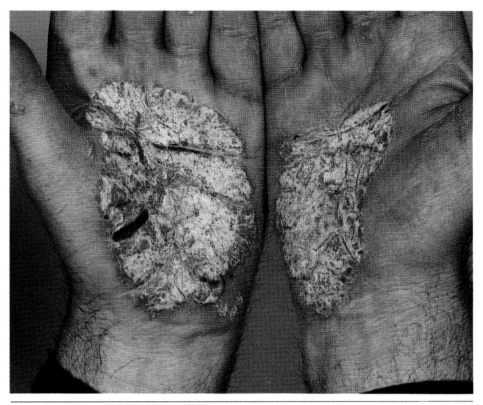

22 Psoriasis of the palms

Patient Profile Fifty-five-year-old male

History For 30 years, widespread psoriasis. For 1 year, lesions on the palms.

Physical Examination On both palms, sharply demarcated, large erythematous patches covered with thick silver-white scales. The lesions are in part fissured and cracked.

Differential Diagnosis Hyperkeratotic eczema of the palms (tylotic eczema)

Clues Sharp demarcation, silver-white scaling, psoriasis lesions elsewhere

Treatment Improved under betamethasone valerate cream with 5% salicylic acid, under plastic occlusion at night. Some resistant areas: intralesional corticosteroids. Later: PUVA therapy with excellent results.

Generalized Pustular Psoriasis Syndrome (von Zumbusch)

This disease is a life-threatening acute medical problem, with sudden onset of fiery red, burning, large areas ("sheets") of skin; fever (sometimes high); generalized weakness; malaise; and high white blood cell count. This relentless, inexorable progression of sheets of fiery erythema spreads over the entire skin surface. Pinpoint pustules appear in the erythematous sheets and the pustules coalesce to form "lakes" of pus (see Figure 23). The nails become involved and separate. Arthropathy occurs in over a third of the patients.

COURSE AND PROGNOSIS

In many patients a complete and spontaneous remission occurs, but relapses are quite frequent; the disease persists for years.

TREATMENT

The patient requires hospitalization. The treatment programs advocated (retinoids, PUVA photochemotherapy, methotrexate, and hydroxyurea) are difficult to evaluate because of the high degree of spontaneous remission. There is a general belief, however, that relapses are less frequent and less severe with these therapies, especially the retinoids such as etretinate (see page 54).

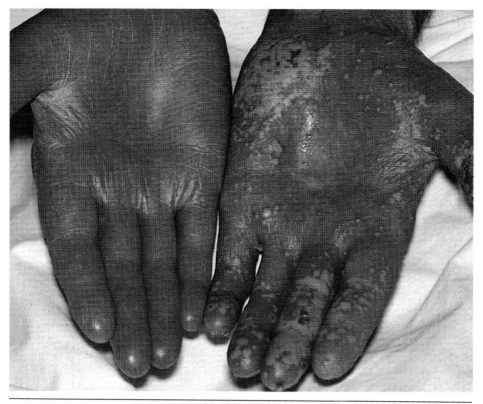

23 Psoriasis pustulosa (von Zumbusch) pustular psoriasis

Patient Profile *Sixty-one-year-old male*

History *For 10 years, generalized pustular eruptions on abdomen, upper legs, and flexor sides of hands and feet. Flares are frequently associated with fever (up to 39°C) and malaise.*

Physical Examination *On the flexor side of the left hand are many pustules, partly arranged in groups and merging. The right hand looks normal except for a slight atrophy of the skin.*

Differential Diagnosis *Pustulosis palmaris et plantaris, follicular impetigo, dyshidrotic eczematous dermatitis with bacterial superinfection, fungal infection*

Laboratory and Special Examinations *Examination for fungi, yeasts, and bacteria: negative. Blood cell count and differential: normal. Histology: pronounced microabscess formation in the epidermis.*

Clues *Sterile pustules on different parts of the body, occasionally psoriasis vulgaris lesions elsewhere, histology*

Treatment *The right hand was treated with betamethasone-17-valerate cream under plastic occlusion with an excellent response; initially the left hand was not treated (paired comparison).*

Palmoplantar Pustulosis

Palmoplantar pustulosis is a chronic, relapsing eruption limited to the palms and soles and characterized by numerous sterile, yellow, deep-seated, small pustules that evolve into dusky-red macules.

EPIDEMIOLOGY AND ETIOLOGY

Incidence Low
Age 50–60 years
Sex More common in females (4:1)
Other Features Patient may or may not have psoriasis or may develop it in other sites (scalp, trunk, etc.)

This disorder may or may not be a variant of psoriasis—studies of a large series of patients showed no increase in the HLA-B13 or -BW17, two antigens that have been found to be associated with psoriasis vulgaris.
Cigarette smoking is a putative exacerbating factor. Stopping smoking, however, may or may not improve the condition.

HISTORY

Duration of Lesions Months
Skin Symptoms Tenderness and burning as new lesions appear and when fissures are present; may interfere with walking or using the hands

PHYSICAL EXAMINATION

Skin Lesions

TYPE Vesicles and pustules in varying stages of evolution, 2.0–5.0 mm, deep-seated, develop into dusky-red macules; present in areas of erythema and scaling
DISTRIBUTION Localized to palms and soles
SITES OF PREDILECTION Thenar and hypothenar, flexor aspects of fingers, heels, and insteps; acral portions of the fingers and toes are usually spared

DIFFERENTIAL DIAGNOSIS

A quite characteristic clinical presentation, but tinea manus and tinea pedis should always be excluded by examination of scales; eczematous dyshidrotic dermatitis (pompholyx) is always pruritic, vesicles are more numerous than pustules, and fissures and secondary infection often occur.

DERMATOPATHOLOGY

Site Epidermis and dermis
Process Edema and exocytosis of mononuclear cells forming a vesicle and later many neutrophils, which form a unilocular pustule that usually extends into the dermis and slightly above the plane of the skin; small spongiform pustules and some acanthosis
Cell Types Mononuclear cells at first and later myriads of neutrophils

PATHOPHYSIOLOGY

A leukotactic factor similar to that found in psoriasis vulgaris has been isolated from the stratum corneum of palmoplantar pustulosis. This could elicit migration to the target tissue of myriads of neutrophils that carry leukotriene B_4, a potent neutrophil chemoattractant.

TREATMENT

The condition is recalcitrant to treatment, but PUVA and etretinate, alone or in combination, are effective but not curative (see page 54 for details). Topical corticosteroids, dithranol, and coal tar are ineffective. Strong corticosteroids under plastic occlusion (e.g., for the night) are often effective but skin atrophy may limit prolonged use.

PROGNOSIS

Persistent for years and characterized by unexplained remissions and exacerbations.

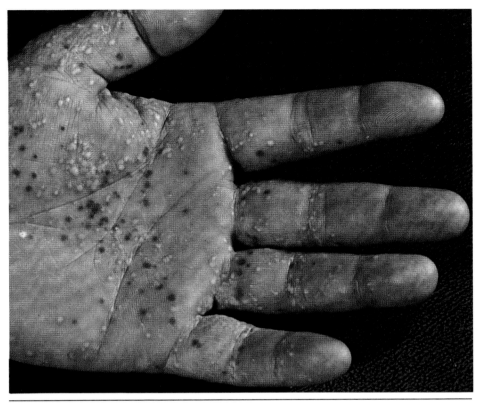

24 Pustulosis palmaris et plantaris

Patient Profile Forty-one-year-old female

History For 1 year, pustular eruptions on flexor sides of hands and feet. No fever, no other complaints.

Physical Examination Disseminated on palm and fingers, many small, deep-seated, yellowish white fresh pustules and brownish pinpoint-sized healing pustules

Differential Diagnosis Psoriasis pustulosa, dyshidrotic eczematous dermatitis with bacterial superinfection, fungal infection

Laboratory and Special Examinations Examination for bacteria, fungi, and yeasts: negative

Clues Deep-seated sterile pustules on palms, brownish discoloration after spontaneous healing; absence of lesions elsewhere

Treatment Corticosteroid cream to which 5% salicylic acid is added, with plastic occlusion at night, brought improvement. Complications: marked atrophy of the skin. Later, less frequent application of steroid ointments and oral aromatic retinoid, 37.5 mg daily. This combination led to a satisfactory result; the formation of new pustules diminished significantly.

IV
Scaling Eruptions
of Unknown Etiology

Seborrheic Dermatitis

This is a common chronic dermatosis characterized by redness and scaling. It occurs in the areas of the skin in which the sebaceous glands are most active, such as the face and scalp, and in the body folds.

EPIDEMIOLOGY

Age Infancy (within the first months), puberty, majority between 20 and 50 years or older

Sex More common in males

Incidence 2% to 5% of the population

Predisposition Factors Often a genetic diathesis, the "seborrheic state," with marked seborrhea and marginal blepharitis. HIV-infected individuals have an increased incidence.

HISTORY

Duration of Lesions Gradual onset

Skin symptoms Pruritus is variable, often increased by perspiration, worse during winter months

PHYSICAL EXAMINATION

Skin Lesions

Type Yellowish-red, often greasy, or white dry scaling macules and papules of varying size (5 to 20 mm), rather sharply marginated. Sticky crusts and fissures are common when external ear, scalp, axillae, groin, and submammary areas are involved (weeping).

Shape Nummular, polycyclic, and even annular on the trunk

Arrangement Scattered, discrete on the face and trunk; diffuse involvement of scalp

Distribution and Major Types of Lesions (based on localization and age)

Hairy areas of head Scalp, eyebrows, eyelashes (blepharitis), beard (follicular orifices); cradle cap

Face The flush areas ("butterfly"), behind ears, on the forehead ("corona seborrheica")

Trunk Simulating lesions of pityriasis rosea, tinea versicolor, or tinea faciale

Body folds Axillae, groin, anogenital area, submammary areas, umbilicus—presents as a diffuse, sharply marginated, brightly erythematous eruption; fissures are common

Genitalia Often with yellow crusts and psoriasiform lesions

DIFFERENTIAL DIAGNOSIS

Psoriasis (the two diseases may be indistinguishable); *dermatophytosis* and *candidiasis,* especially in intertriginous seborrheic dermatitis (potassium hydroxide examination and cultures will help); *histiocytosis X* (occurs in infants, usually associated with perifollicular purpura); *acrodermatitis enteropathica; lupus erythematosus* (especially for facial—parasasal—lesions biopsy is rarely necessary); *pemphigus foliaceus; glucagonoma*

DERMATOPATHOLOGY

Site Epidermis

Process Focal parakeratosis, with few pyknotic neutrophils, moderate acanthosis, spongiosis (intercellular edema), nonspecific inflammation of the dermis. The most characteristic feature is neutrophils at the tips of the dilated follicular openings, which appear as crusts/scales

PATHOPHYSIOLOGY

No etiologic organism has been proved, yet pyogenic infection is often present. Experimental inoculations have not been successful in producing seborrheic dermatitis. *Pityrosporon ovale* plays a role in the pathogenesis of some patients. Diet, alcohol, emotions could play some role. Seborrheic dermatitis-like lesions are seen in nutritional deficiencies such as zinc deficiency (as a result of intravenous alimentation) and experimental niacin deficiency, and in Parkinson's disease (including drug-induced).

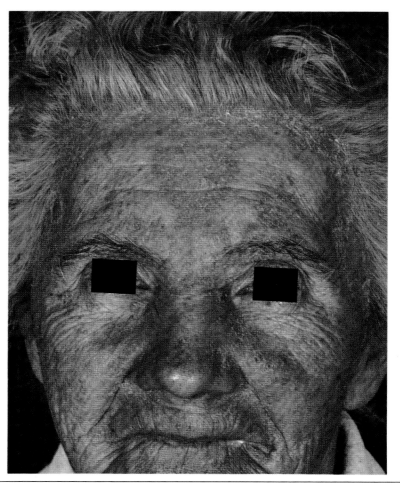

25 Seborrheic dermatitis

Patient Profile Seventy-eight-year-old female

History For 2 months, a rash on the face

Physical Examination Erythematous scaling lesions on the forehead, especially along the hairline, in the eyebrows, in the nasolabial folds. The scales are yellow. Yellowish scaling of the scalp.

Clues Erythematous yellow scaling lesions with typical localization; absence of pruritus

Treatment Rapid improvement using 1% hydrocortisone cream

COURSE AND PROGNOSIS

Recurrences and remissions, especially on the scalp, may be associated with alopecia in severe cases. Infantile and adolescent seborrheic dermatitis disappear with age. Seborrheic erythroderma (Leiner's disease) may occur.

TREATMENT

Scalp Removal of crusts with 2% to 3% salicylic acid in olive oil is essential; shampoos containing selenium sulfide or zinc pyrithione or tar; topical vioform-hydrocortisone lotion or betamethasone valerate lotion following one of these medicated shampoos for more severe cases.

Face Hydrocortisone acetate cream, 1% or 2.5% bid. Avoid prolonged fluorinated corticosteroids because of side effects telangiectasis, erythema, and perioral dermatitis). Creams containing ketoconazole or 3% sulfur and 2% salicylic acid are alternatives to topical corticosteroids and should be used for chronic resistant lesions, especially on the face and chest.

Intertriginous Areas Castellani's paint in oozing dermatitis of the body folds (often very effective)

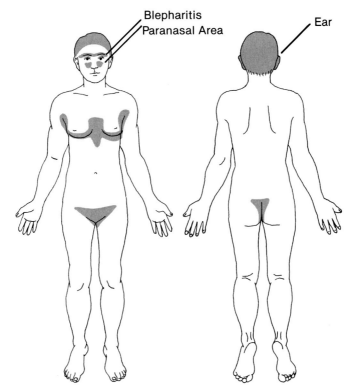

Figure VI
Seborrheic Dermatitis

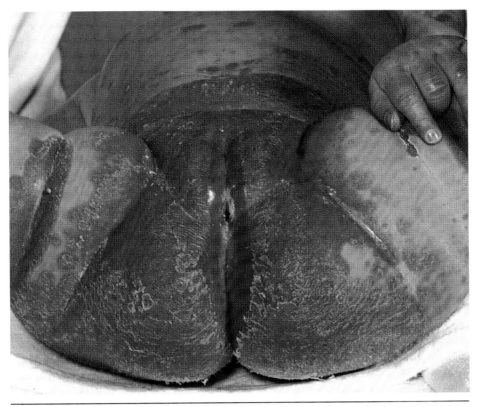

26 Seborrheic dermatitis in an infant

Patient Profile Five-month-old female infant

History For 8 weeks, an eruption that started on the buttocks and spread to the trunk, scalp, and retroauricular area

Physical Examination Erythematous, scaling, confluent macules in the diaper region and skin folds; disseminated, erythematous, scaling macules next to the confluent regions, around the umbilicus, in the axillae, laterally on the neck, and behind the ears. Oily scaling of the scalp. Lesions are sharply demarcated.

Differential Diagnosis Candidiasis, atopic eczema, psoriasis

Laboratory Examinations Mycologic examination: negative.

Clues Localization in body folds and on scalp, absence of pruritus, negative mycology

Treatment Rapid improvement with topical sulfur and topical corticosteroids

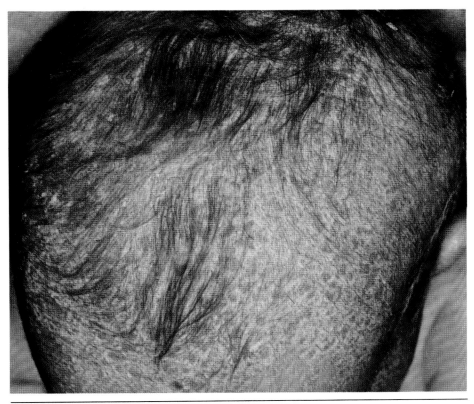

27 Seborrheic dermatitis of infants (cradle cap)

Patient Profile *Two-month-old male infant*

History *Since birth, an eruption of the scalp and cheeks, later also in skin folds. No pruritus.*

Physical Examination *Diffusely involving the scalp, yellow oily scales and a few scattered erythematous round patches; also erythematous scaling eruptions around the umbilicus, in the inguinal folds, and on the scrotum*

Clues *Nature and distribution of the eruption, no pruritus*

Treatment *Scalp: 5% coal tar solution and 5% sulfur in a cream base. Skin folds: 2% sulfur cream. Rapid improvement occurred.*

This exanthematous, maculopapular, red, scaling (Latin *pityriasis,* "scaling") eruption occurs largely on the trunk and is probably caused by an infectious agent, most likely a virus.

EPIDEMIOLOGY

Age Ten to thirty-five years
Incidence Two percent of dermatologic outpatients

HISTORY

Duration of Lesions Days. A "herald" patch (see Figure 28, two o'clock position) precedes the exanthematous phase by 1 to 2 weeks. The exanthe-matous phase develops over a period of a week.

Skin Symptoms Pruritus—absent, mild, or severe

PHYSICAL EXAMINATION

Skin Lesions

TYPE

Herald plaque (80 percent of patients); 2-to 5-cm, bright red, fine scale

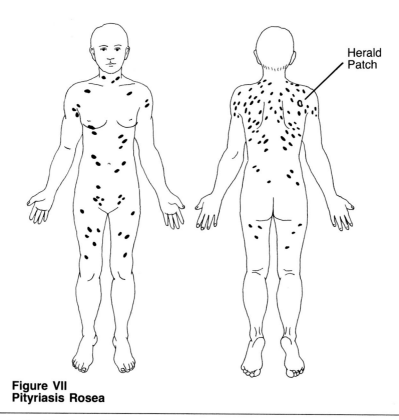

Herald
Patch

Figure VII
Pityriasis Rosea

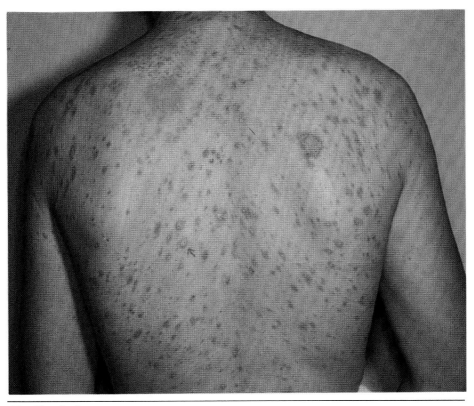

28 Pityriasis rosea

Patient Profile Thirty-six-year-old female

History For 3 weeks, a nonpruritic rash on the trunk and upper arms. Started with one single patch on right scapula. General condition is good, no fever, no drug history.

Physical Examination Scattered over the back and the shoulders are ovoid erythematous patches with somewhat elevated borders, on the inner margin of which fine scaling is seen. Their long axes are in the lines of cleavage of the skin. On the right scapula is the primary patch (larger than the others).

Differential Diagnosis Secondary syphilis (see Figure 100), guttate psoriasis, drug eruption (captopril), nummular eczematous dermatitis

Laboratory and Special Examinations Direct microscopy for fungi. BSR, blood cell counts and serologic tests for syphilis: all normal or negative.

Clues Ovoid-shaped "medallion like" patches, arranged according to the lines of cleavage of the skin. Face and distal parts of extremities unaffected.

Treatment Cleared spontaneously in 4 weeks. No recurrence.

Exanthem: fine-scaling macules and papules with *typical marginal collarette* (Figure 29)

COLOR   Dull pink or tawny (exanthem)
SHAPE   Oval
ARRANGEMENT   Scattered discrete lesions
DISTRIBUTION   Characteristic pattern of lesions—the long axes of the lesions follow the lines of cleavage in a "Christmas tree" distribution (see Figures VII and 28). Lesions usually confined to trunk and proximal aspects of the arms and legs.

DIFFERENTIAL DIAGNOSIS

Drug eruptions by history, i.e., captopril, *secondary syphilis* (serology always positive; be sure to obtain an STS to rule out secondary syphilis), *guttate psoriasis* (no marginal collarette), erythema chronicum migrans with secondary lesions.

DERMATOPATHOLOGY

Nonspecific

COURSE

Spontaneous remission in 2 to 6 weeks or less. If the eruption persists for over 6 weeks, a skin biopsy should be done to rule out parapsoriasis.

TREATMENT

Pruritis may be controlled by UVB treatment if this is begun in the first week of the eruption. The protocol is five consecutive exposures starting with 80% of the minimum erythema dose and increasing 17% each exposure.

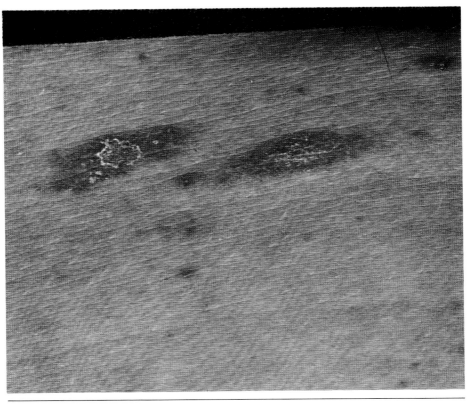

29 Pityriasis rosea

Close-up view of two ovoid red macules with delicate white scaling collar and long axes in the lines of cleavage of the skin

V

Disorders of

Sebaceous Glands

Acne Vulgaris (Common Acne) and Acne Cystica

Acne is a chronic inflammation of the pilosebaceous units of certain areas (face and trunk) that occurs in adolescence and manifests as comedones, papules, nodules, cysts, or papulopustules, often but not always followed by pitted or hypertrophic scars.

EPIDEMIOLOGY AND ETIOLOGY

Age Ten to seventeen in females; 14 to 19 in males

Sex More severe (39 percent of patients) in males than females

Race Lower incidence in Orientals and blacks

Occupation Exposure to acnegenic mineral oils

Drugs Lithium, hydantoin, systemic corticosteroids may cause exacerbation

Genetic Aspects Multifactorial; severe acne associated with XYY syndrome

Other Factors Endocrine (see Pathophysiology) and emotional stress (school, social problems) can definitely cause exacerbations. Pressure on skin by leaning face on the hands is a very important factor causing exacerbation. Acne is not caused by chocolate, fatty foods, or, in fact, any kinds of foods.

HISTORY

Duration of Lesions Months

Season Worse in fall and winter

Symptoms Pain in lesions (especially nodulocystic type)

PHYSICAL EXAMINATION

Skin Lesions

TYPE

Comedo—open (blackheads, Figure 31) or closed (whiteheads)

Papules (Figure 30) with (red) or without inflammation

Nodules, noduloulcerative lesions, or cysts, 2 to 5 cm in diameter (Figure 32)

Scars—atrophic depressed (often pitted) or hypertrophic (keloid) scars

Seborrhea of the face and scalp is often present

SHAPE Round; nodules may coalesce to form linear mounds

ARRANGEMENT Isolated single lesion (e.g., nodule) or scattered discrete lesions (papules, cysts, nodules)

SITES OF PREDILECTION Face, neck, upper arms, trunk

DIFFERENTIAL DIAGNOSIS

Persistent acne in a hirsute female with irregular or no menses is an indication for a search for hypersecretion of androgens, plasma testosterone, and/or dehydroepiandrosterone (e.g., polycystic ovarian syndrome). Also, recalcitrant acne can be related to partial 11- or 12-hydroxylase block.

PATHOPHYSIOLOGY

The lesions of acne (comedones) are the result of complex effects of hormones (androgens) and bacteria *(Propionibacterium acnes)* in the pilosebaceous unit. Androgens stimulate sebaceous glands to produce larger amounts of sebum; bacteria contain lipase that converts lipid into fatty acids. Both sebum and fatty acids cause a sterile inflammatory response in the pilosebaceous unit; this results in hyperkeratinization of the lining of the follicle with resultant desquamation. The enlarged follicular lumen contains this inspissated keratin and lipid debris (the whitehead). When the follicle has a portal of entry at the skin, the semisolid mass protrudes, forming a plug (the blackhead). The black color is due to oxidation of tyrosine to melanin by tyrosinase contained in the follicular orifice. The distended follicle may break and the contents (sebum, lipid, fatty acids, keratin, etc.) enter the dermis, provoking a foreign-body response (papule, pustule, nodule). Rupture plus intense inflammation leads to scars.

COURSE

Acne may persist in women to age 35.

TREATMENT

Mild

Topical antibiotics (clindamycin, erythromycin)

Benzoyl peroxide gels (2, 5 or 10%)

Topical retinoids (vitamin A acid) are

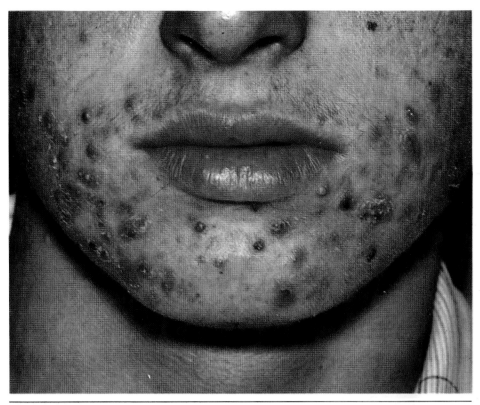

30 Acne vulgaris

Patient Profile Eighteen-year-old boy

History For 3 years, steadily increasing number of "pimples" on face

Physical Examination Papules, pustules, and a few comedones on cheeks and chin. Oily seborrhea.

Differential Diagnosis Folliculitis

Laboratory and Special Examinations Bacterial culture: Propionibacterium acnes.

Clues Age, location, clinical appearance

Treatment One percent clindamycin lotion and 5% benzoyl peroxide gel. Much improved in 6 weeks.

effective, but require detailed instructions and gradual increases in concentration. Improvement occurs over a period of months (2–5) and may be even longer for noninflamed comedones. For most patients, start with Retin-A 0.01% gel and increase after 1 month to 0.025% applied nightly after washing with a mild soap. Topical antibiotics are applied during the day.

Severe

Oral antibiotics added to the above—minocycline, 50 to 100 mg bid—is probably the most effective.
In females, severe acne can be controlled with high doses of oral estrogens combined with progesterone. Cerebrovascular disorders are a serious risk, however.

Oral 13-*cis*-retinoic acid (Accutane) is highly effective for cystic acne. In general, however, only persons who have extensive experience in using Accutane should prescribe it. As retinoids are teratogenic in females, it is necessary that female patients have pretreatment pregnancy test and they must be on oral contraceptives at least 1 month prior to beginning treatment, throughout treatment, and for 1 month after treatment is discontinued. Furthermore, a patient must have a negative serum pregnancy test within the prior 2 weeks before beginning treatment. Dosage: 0.5–1 mg/kg/day with meals for a 15- to 20-week course, which is usually adequate. About 30% of patients require two 4-month courses with a 2-month rest period in between. Careful monitoring of the blood is necessary during therapy, especially in patients with elevated blood triglycerides before therapy is begun.

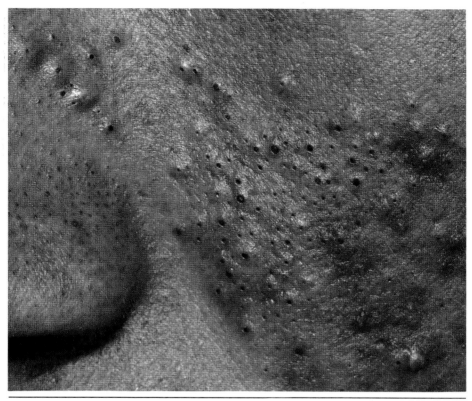

31 Acne vulgaris

Patient Profile Twenty-year-old male

History For 5 years, acne on face

Physical Examination Many blackheads (open comedones) and a few whiteheads (closed comedones), some papules and pustules

Treatment Vitamin A acid (0.05 to 0.1%) in a lotion; subsequent removal of comedones with a comedone extractor. Later, 1% clindamycin lotion and 5% salicylic acid, 5% resorcinol in O/W cream. Much improved in 3 months.

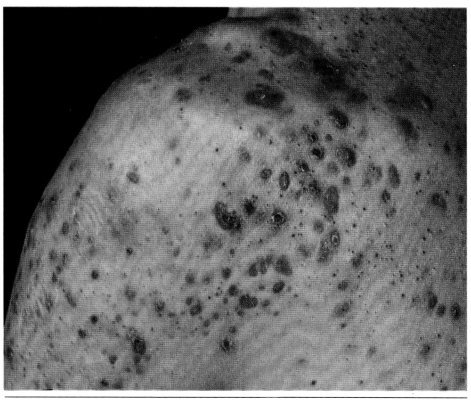

32 Acne cystica

Patient Profile Twenty-two-year-old male

History For 7 years, acne, primarily on the face; later, chiefly on the back

Physical Examination On the shoulder and upper part of the back, many purple-red, papular to nodular infiltrates and numerous blackheads

Differential Diagnosis Folliculitis

Laboratory and Special Examinations *Bacterial cultures:* Propionibacterium acnes.

Clues *Indurated, partly coalescing, purple-red lesions; location; age*

Treatment *Oral tetracycline, 1 g daily; later, 0.5 g. Topically, 10% salicylic acid and 10% resorcinol in O/W cream; subsequently, 5 to 10% benzoyl peroxide gel. Much improved in 3 months. Isotretinoin (Accutane) orally as an alternative.*

Rosacea

Rosacea (Latin, "like roses") is a chronic acneform inflammation of the pilosebaceous units of the face, coupled with a peculiar increased reactivity of capillaries to heat, leading to flushing and telangiectasia.

EPIDEMIOLOGY AND ETIOLOGY

Age Thirty to fifty years
Sex Females predominantly
Race Celtic peoples (Skin Phototypes I and II); less frequent in pigmented (brown and black) peoples
Other Factors Patients have periodic reddening of the face (flushing) with increase in skin temperature in response to heat stimuli in the mouth (hot liquids); alcohol is a definite factor in rosacea, possibly by its "flushing" effect.

HISTORY

Duration of Lesions Days, weeks
Skin Symptoms Flushing; papular and papulopustular lesions may be tender

PHYSICAL EXAMINATION

Skin Lesions

TYPE

Telangiectasia (Figure 33)
Papules (2 to 3 mm), papulopustules [the pustule (Figure 34) is often minute on the "crest" of the papule]
Nodules (Figure 34)
No comedones

COLOR Rose-red facies, papules and nodules (Figures 33 and 34)
SHAPE Papules and nodules are round, dome-shaped
ARRANGEMENT Scattered discrete lesions

DISTRIBUTION Characteristic is a symmetrical localization on the face (cheeks, chin, forehead, nose) and, rarely, neck
Eye lesions Blepharitis, conjunctivitis, and episcleritis. Rosacea keratitis (33 percent) is a serious problem as corneal ulcers may develop. An ophthalmologist should follow the patient with eye involvement.

DIFFERENTIAL DIAGNOSIS

The differential diagnosis of flushing will include carcinoid syndrome and systemic lupus erythematosus, but the sine qua non of the diagnosis of rosacea are the small papules and papulopustules.

COURSE

Prolonged. Recurrences are common. After a few years the disease tends to disappear spontaneously. Men may develop rhinophyma, which is successfully treated by surgery.

TREATMENT

Marked reduction or elimination of alcoholic and hot beverages.
Tetracycline or erythromycin 250 mg tid for 1 week, then bid and gradually reduced to daily doses.
Topical 0.75% metronidazole is a new, very effective treatment.
Topical antibiotics are somewhat effective.
Emotional stress may be a definite factor and should be emphasized to the patient.

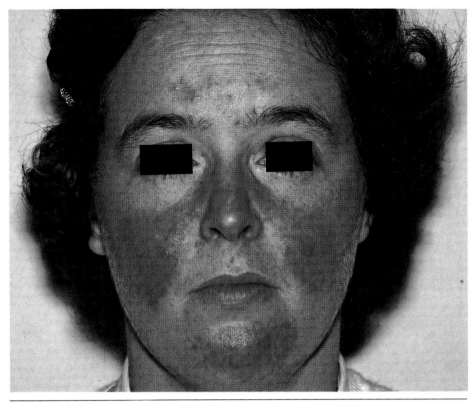

33 Rosacea

Patient Profile Forty-six-year-old female

History For 14 years, red patches and "pimples" on face. No other complaints

Physical Examination On the forehead above the nose, on both cheeks, the nose, and the chin, nonscaling erythematous areas, slightly indurated, sharply demarcated. Several papular infiltrates and a few small pustules.

Differential Diagnosis Lupus erythematosus

Laboratory and Special Examinations Bacterial culture: sterile. Histology: normal epidermis. In the dermis, dense cellular infiltrates, mainly consisting of lymphocytes, partly arranged about the sebaceous glands. A few foci of epitheloid cells and one Langhans giant cell. Immunofluorescence: negative.

Treatment Cleared in 6 weeks with oral tetracycline, 1 g daily for 3 weeks; later, 0.5 g; maintenance, 0.250 g. No recurrence with this regimen.

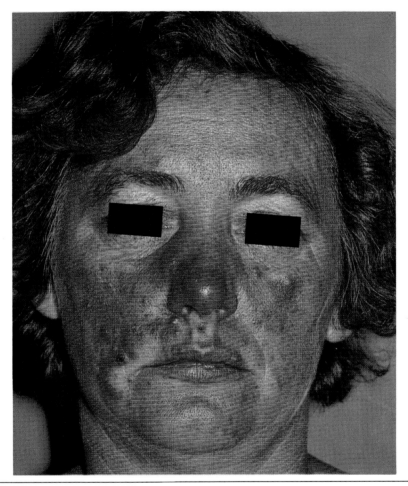

34 Rosacea

Patient Profile Fifty-three-year-old female

History For 6 months, red inflammatory patches and "pimples" on the face. No other complaints.

Physical Examination On the cheeks and the nose, slightly indurated erythematous areas with many papules and pustules. No comedones.

Differential Diagnosis Lupus erythematosus, acne, folliculitis

Laboratory and Special Examinations Bacterial culture: sterile. Histology: rosacea (see Figure 33).

Clues Age, location, appearance, absence of comedones. Presence of papulopustules argues against lupus erythematosus.

Treatment Cleared with oral tetracycline, 1 g daily, and remained well under 2.50 mg maintenance. Recurrences after discontinuation.

VI
Disorders of Hair

Alopecia areata (AA) is a localized loss of hair in round or oval areas without any visible inflammation on the scalp skin or skin symptoms. All of the hair of the body may eventually be lost (alopecia totalis).

EPIDEMIOLOGY AND ETIOLOGY

Age Young adults (under 25 years); children are frequently affected
Sex Equal in both sexes, although male/female ratio is 2 : 1 in Italy and Spain
Race In every race; 20 percent give a family history
Other Factors Not a sign of any multisystem disease, but may be associated with other autoimmune disorders such as vitiligo, familial multiendocrine syndrome, and thyroid disease (Hashimoto's disease). Emotional problems, especially life crises, can precipitate an attack.

HISTORY

Duration of Lesions Gradual over weeks
Skin Symptoms None, tenderness may occur early

PHYSICAL EXAMINATION

Skin Lesions None, possible erythema
Hair Alopecia occasionally with diagnostic broken-off stubby hairs called *exclamation point hairs*
ARRANGEMENT Scattered discrete areas of alopecia, or confluent (total loss of hair)
DISTRIBUTION Localized (to scalp or eyelids or cheek) or generalized with total loss (alopecia totalis)
SITES OF PREDILECTION Scalp, eyebrows, eyelashes, pubic hair, beard

Nails Dystrophic changes (20 percent): fine stippling like "hammered brass"

DERMATOPATHOLOGY

Follicles, which are reduced in size, arrested in anagen IV and lie high in the dermis; perifollicular lymphocytic infiltrate with degenerative changes in the blood vessels that lead to the hair papilla. Increase of telogen hair from normal (less than 20 percent) to 25 to 40 percent

COURSE

If occurring after puberty, 80 percent of patients regrow hair. Total alopecia is rare. Following the first episode of hair loss about 33 percent completely regrow the hair within a year. Recurrences of alopecia, however, are frequent. Repeated attacks, nail changes, and total alopecia before puberty are poor prognostic signs.

TREATMENT

Topical clobetasol proprionate ointment used for 6 weeks only as skin atrophy can occur.
Minoxidil lotion used for months may be partially effective in 30 percent of patients.
Wigs are very satisfactory, especially for women.
Avoid systemic corticosteroids.

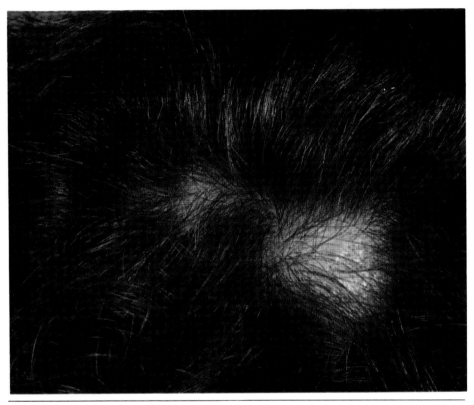

35 Alopecia areata

Patient Profile Forty-five-year-old female

History For 6 weeks, two circular bald patches on scalp. No pruritus, no other complaints.

Physical Examination On the crown of the scalp, two sharply outlined patches with subtotal hair loss. The largest patch is 3 cm in diameter. Except for mild dandruff, there is no abnormal scaling or erythema. On close inspection the follicles seem intact and there is no atrophy.

Differential Diagnosis Tinea capitis, cicatricial alopecia, secondary syphilis, chronic discoid lupus erythematosus

Laboratory and Special Examinations Examination for fungi and serologic tests for syphilis: negative. Histology: round cell infiltrate around lower half of hair follicles. Hair morphology: predominantly dystrophic hairs.

Clues Rapidly developing circumscribed round or ovoid patches of hair loss, without signs of inflammation, and intact follicles

VII

Disorders of
the Dermis and
Dermal-Epidermal
Interface

This acute or chronic inflammation of the skin and mucous membrane has characteristic flat-topped (Latin *planus,* "flat"), violaceous, shiny, pruritic papules, and milky-white papules in the mouth.

EPIDEMIOLOGY AND ETIOLOGY

Age Thirty to sixty years
Sex Females more than males
Other Factors The etiology is unknown. Severe emotional stress can precipitate an attack.

HISTORY

Duration of Lesions Acute (days) or insidious onset in weeks

Symptoms

SKIN Pruritus, which may be severe or absent
MUCOUS MEMBRANE Painful, especially when ulcers present

PHYSICAL EXAMINATION

Skin Lesions

TYPE Papules, 1 to 10 mm, shiny
COLOR Violaceous, with white lines (Wickham's striae, Figure 36) seen best with hand lens after mineral oil
SHAPE Polygonal or oval
ARRANGEMENT Grouped, linear (isomorphic phenomenon), annular, or disseminated scattered discrete lesions
DISTRIBUTION Wrists (flexor, see Figure 36), lumbar region, eyelids, shins (thicker, hyperkeratotic lesions), and scalp
Mucous Membrane Forty to sixty percent. See Figure 37.
SITES OF PREDILECTION Buccal mucosa, tongue, lips
LESIONS Milky-white papules, with white lacework on the buccal mucosa. Carcinoma may develop in mouth lesions (see Figure 37).

Hair and Nails

SCALP Atrophic scalp skin with alopecia
NAILS (10 PERCENT) Destruction of the nail fold and nail bed, especially the large toe

DIFFERENTIAL DIAGNOSIS

Drug eruption caused by contact with chemicals used in color developing. *Chloroquine* given orally. A biopsy is necessary in most cases, but the identification by Wickham's striae is quite specific.

DERMATOPATHOLOGY

Site Epidermis and dermis
Process Inflammation with hyperkeratosis, increased granular layer, irregular acanthosis, liquefaction degeneration of the basal cell layer, and bandlike mononuclear infiltrate that hugs the epidermis

COURSE

Spontaneous resolution in weeks is possible; lesions may also persist for years, especially on the shins and in the mouth.

TREATMENT

Topical corticosteroids with occlusion.
Oral prednisone is rarely used, and only in short courses.
PUVA photochemotherapy may be substituted for oral prednisone in generalized or resistant cases.
Oral retinoids are helpful for erosive lichen planus of the mouth.

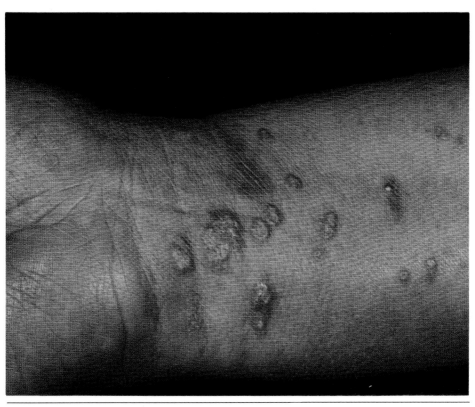

36 Lichen planus

Patient Profile *Fifty-year-old female homemaker*

History *A pruritic eruption on arms and back for 6 months*

Physical Examination *Flat papules on the right wrist, some of which are coalescent and some are isolated. Color is violaceous, with pearly lines and central umbilication. Severe pruritus; no lesions in the mouth.*

Differential Diagnosis *Papular eczema*

Dermatopathology *Hyperkeratosis, local thickening of the stratum granulosum, acanthosis, rete ridges irregular with partial "sawtooth" appearance, fuzzy demarcation between epidermis and dermis. Bandlike infiltration, with a sharp lower border, of the dermis by lymphocytes.*

Clues *Wickham's striae, histopathology*

Treatment *Oral prednisone; topically, cream with 0.1% triamcinolone acetonide. Under gradually diminishing oral dosage of prednisone, only slow improvement. After 2 and 5 years, typical recurrences.*

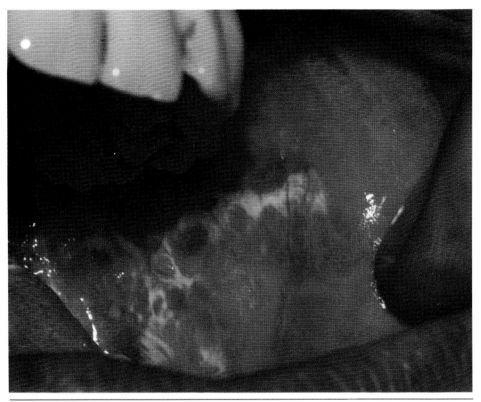

37 Lichen planus of the mouth

Patient Profile Thirty-six-year-old male

History For 3 months, white and occasionally painful lesions on the buccal mucosa

Physical Examination On both sides, the buccal mucosa shows irregularly marginated, white areas which are not elevated or indurated. The surface is smooth and the lesions are surrounded by an erythematous zone. On the flexor surfaces of the wrists are a few pruritic papules.

Differential Diagnosis Candidiasis, leukoplakia, oral hairy leukoplakia

Laboratory and Special Examinations Biopsy: lichen planus. Direct microscopy and culture for yeasts: negative for Candida.

Clues Two-dimensional, white, linear or reticular lesions on the mucosa; presence of typical lichen planus lesions on the skin; histology

Treatment Much improved under topical treatment with 0.1% triamcinolone acetonide and 0.05% retinoic acid in Orabase, and subsequently intralesional corticosteroids

Granuloma Annulare

This disease is a self-limited chronic inflammation of the dermis that exhibits papules in an annular arrangement.

EPIDEMIOLOGY AND ETIOLOGY

Age Children and young adults
Sex Female/male ratio 2 : 1
Other Factors Etiology is unknown. The lesions are sometimes indistinguishable from necrobiosis lipoidica. In generalized granuloma annulare, diabetes mellitus has been reported.

HISTORY

Duration of Lesions Weeks, months
Skin Symptoms Usually asymptomatic, rarely pruritic

PHYSICAL EXAMINATION

Skin Lesions

TYPE

Firm dermal papules 1 to 5 cm, rare epidermal change* (see Figure 38)
Nodules, subcutaneous

COLOR Skin-colored, erythematous, violaceous
SHAPE Dome-shaped, annular
ARRANGEMENT Complete circle (annular) or half-circle (arciform)
DISTRIBUTION Isolated lesion (Figure 38), multiple lesions in certain regions, or generalized (older patients)

SITES OF PREDILECTION

Dermal papules Dorsa of hands, fingers, feet, extensor aspects of arms and legs, trunk

Subcutaneous nodules Palms, legs, buttocks, scalp

DIFFERENTIAL DIAGNOSIS

Papular lesions (necrobiosis, lipoidica, papular sarcoid, lichen planus, lymphocytic infiltrate of Lessner); subcutaneous nodules (rheumatoid nodules)

DERMATOPATHOLOGY

Site Dermis or subcutaneous tissue
Process Foci of chronic inflammation in subpapillary plexus of blood vessels with incomplete and reversible necrosis (necrobiosis) of connective tissue surrounded by a wall of palisading histiocytes and multinucleated giant cells

COURSE

The disease disappears in 75 percent of patients in 2 years, but recurrences are common (40 percent).

TREATMENT

Intralesional triamcinolone acetonide, 5 mg/ml, or topical corticosteroids with occlusion; corticosteroids incorporated in tape are somewhat useful

---

*So-called perforating granuloma annular

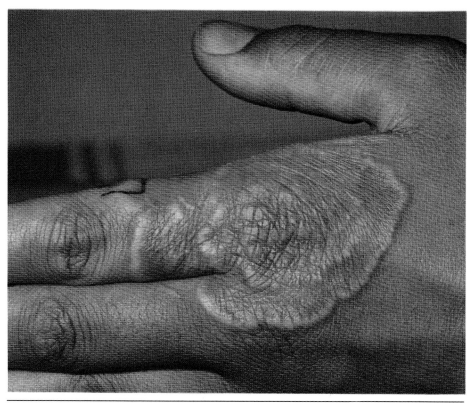

38 Granuloma annulare

Patient Profile Fifty-nine-year-old bartender

History For several years, a gradually expanding growth on the left hand. Patient had mild diabetes.

Physical Examination On the back of the left hand and fingers II and III, confluent, pearly-white, firm papules forming two rings 1 and 5 cm in diameter

Differential Diagnosis Tinea manus

Laboratory and Special Examinations Mycologic examination: negative

Sarcoidosis

Sarcoidosis is a chronic granulomatous inflammation in young adults, affecting diverse organs, but presents primarily as skin lesions, eye lesions, bilateral hilar lymphadenopathy, and pulmonary infiltration.

EPIDEMIOLOGY AND ETIOLOGY

Age Under 40 years (range: 12 to 70 years)
Sex Equal incidence in males and females
Race All races. In the United States and South Africa, much more frequent in blacks and frequent in Scandinavia
Other Factors The disease occurs worldwide, and there is no clue as to the etiology. The disease can occur in families.

HISTORY

Duration of Lesions Days (presenting as acute erythema nodosum) or months (presenting as pulmonary infiltrate discovered in routine chest radiography)
Skin Symptoms May be painful (erythema nodosum)
Constitutional Symptoms Fever, fatigue, weight loss, arrhythmia
Systems Review Enlarged parotids, cardiac dyspnea, neuropathy, kidney stones, uveitis, arthralgia (with erythema nodosum)

PHYSICAL EXAMINATION

Skin Lesions

TYPE AND COLOR

Erythema nodosum syndrome (see page 130)
Purple infiltrated plaques (see Figure 49)
Lupus pernio—violaceous, soft, doughy nodules on the nose, cheek, and earlobes
Multiple maculopapular lesions, 0.5 to 1.0 cm, yellowish-brown
"Scar sarcoidosis"—translucent purple-red nodules occurring in an old scar

SHAPE Annular, polycyclic (see Figure 39), serpiginous
ARRANGEMENT Scattered discrete lesions (maculopapular and nodular types) and diffuse infiltration (lupus pernio)

DISTRIBUTION

Plaques Extremities, buttocks
Papular Face, extremities
Erythema nodosum Legs
Lupus pernio Nose, cheek, and earlobes
"Scar sarcoidosis" Knees
Miscellaneous Findings Lymphadenopathy, hepatosplenomegaly, cardiac arrhythmias, uveitis, enlarged parotid; may involve only the skin, as in Figure 39

RADIOGRAPHIC STUDIES

Ninety percent of patients: hilar lymphadenopathy, pulmonary infiltrate

DIAGNOSIS

Tissue biopsy of skin or lymph nodes is the best criterion for diagnosis of sarcoidosis.

LABORATORY AND SPECIAL EXAMINATIONS

Dermatopathology

Site: dermis. Large islands of epitheloid cells with a few giant cells, and lymphocytes, so-called naked tubercles
Kveim–Siltzbach Test (Antigen prepared from human sarcoid spleen or lymph nodes) Material injected and resulting papule excised in 6 weeks; positive in 50 to 80 percent, especially in untreated patients with skin lesions and lymphadenopathy. Not in common use; antigen not readily available.

Blood Chemistry

Increase in serum angiotensin-converting enzyme (ACE)
Hypergammaglobulinemia
Hypercalcemia

TREATMENT

Systemic corticosteroids for active ocular disease, active pulmonary disease, cardiac arrhythmia, CNS

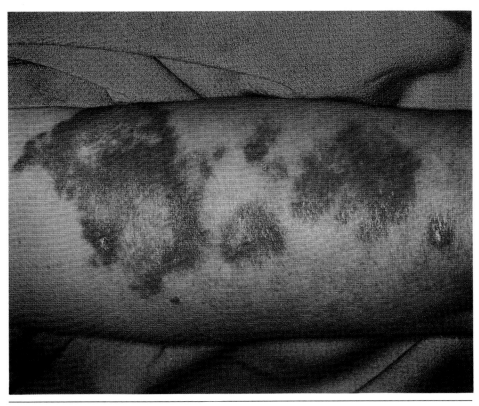

39 Sarcoidosis

Patient Profile   Forty-six-year-old female homemaker

History   For several years, brown violaceous infiltrations of the left upper arm

Physical Examination   On the left upper arm, firm, irregularly demarcated, brownish-violet infiltrated patches. Normal sensitivity to touch and temperature.

Differential Diagnosis   Tuberculosis cutis, leprosy

Laboratory and Special Examinations   Biopsy: sarcoidosis. X-ray of chest: slightly enlarged hilar nodes, lungs normal. X-ray of bones: normal. Ophthalmologic examination: negative. Tuberculin test: negative. Kveim reagent not available.

Clues   Clinical picture, typical histopathology, absence of leprosy

Treatment   Betamethasone-17-valerate cream under occlusion. Gradual disappearance.

involvement, or hypercalcemia. Chloroquine is helpful if disfiguring skin involvement is the major problem.

For skin lesions, topical corticosteroids under plastic dressings (see Figure 39).

VIII
Bullous Diseases

Pemphigus vulgaris is a serious acute or chronic, bullous, autoimmune disease of skin and mucous membranes that is potentially fatal unless treated with immunosuppressive agents.

EPIDEMIOLOGY AND ETIOLOGY

Age Forty to sixty years
Sex Equal incidence in males and females
Race Jewish and Mediterranean people, high incidence
Etiology Autoimmune disorder; a pemphigus foliaceous-like syndrome can be induced by D-penicillamine, and captopril

HISTORY

Duration of Lesions Pemphigus vulgaris starts usually in oral mucosa, and months may elapse before skin lesions occur; these may be localized for 6 to 12 months, following which generalized bullae then occur.
Skin Symptoms No pruritus; painful and tender mouth lesions may prevent adequate food intake
Constitutional Symptoms Weakness, malaise, weight loss (if prolonged mouth involvement)
System Review Epistaxis, hoarseness, dysphagia

PHYSICAL EXAMINATION

Skin Lesions

TYPE

Vesicles and bullae (Figure 40) flaccid (flabby), easily ruptured, and weeping, arising on normal skin
Erosions, crusts
COLOR Skin-colored
SHAPE Round or oval
ARRANGEMENT Randomly scattered discrete lesions
DISTRIBUTION Localized (e.g., to mouth) or generalized with a random pattern (see Figure VIII)
SITES OF PREDILECTION Scalp, face, chest, axillae, groin, umbilicus

Mucous Membranes Bullae rarely seen, erosions of mouth and nose, pharynx and larynx, vagina

DIFFERENTIAL DIAGNOSIS

Can be a difficult, subtle problem, especially if only mouth lesions present. Biopsy of the skin and mucous membrane and direct immunofluorescence are usually able to confirm a high index of suspicion.

LABORATORY AND SPECIAL EXAMINATIONS

Dermatopathology Light microscopy (select early small bulla): (1) loss of intercellular bridges in lower part of epidermis, leading to (2) acantholysis (separation of keratinocytes) and to (3) bulla which is split just *above* the basal cell layer
Immunofluorescence (IF) Direct IF staining reveals IgG and often C3 deposited at the site of the primary lesion in *the intercellular substance.* Antibodies in the serum by indirect immunofluorescence.

PATHOPHYSIOLOGY

A loss of the normal cell-to-cell adhesion in the epidermis occurs as a result of circulatory antibodies of the IgG class; these antibodies bind to the cell surface protein of the epidermis.

COURSE

The disease inexorably progresses to death unless treated aggressively with immunosuppressive agents. The mortality has been markedly reduced since treatment has become available.

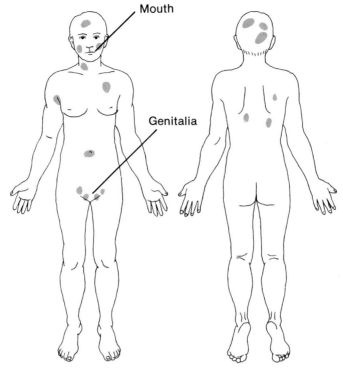

Mouth

Genitalia

Figure VIII
Pemphigus Vulgaris

TREATMENT

Prednisone, 1.0 to 2.0 mg/kg in divided doses until lesions have cleared; then a single daily dose can be given reducing 5 to 10 mg/per week until 40 mg, at which time alternate-day therapy is begun (40 mg/0 mg). The alternate-day dose is then gradually reduced. Prednisone is often combined with other immunosuppressive agents.

Immunosuppressive drugs (azathioprine or cyclophosphamide or methotrexate) are usually started when the prednisone doses are being reduced.

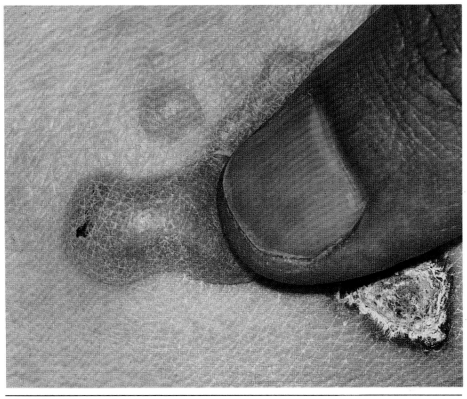

40 Pemphigus vulgaris

Patient Profile Seventy-one-year-old female

History For 6 weeks, rapidly progressive, generalized bullous eruption on trunk and extremities. No other complaints.

Physical Examination Large number of tense bullae on normal and nonhealing erosions and crusts. The blisters extend on pressure with the finger (Nikolsky's sign). The normal skin near the blisters shows easy epidermolysis by drawing the finger with firm pressure over the surface (Nikolsky's sign).

Differential Diagnosis Bullous pemphigoid, bullous dermatitis herpetiformis, drug eruption, erythema multiforme

Laboratory and Special Examinations Histology: intraepidermal blister due to acantholysis. Immunofluorescence: deposits of immunoglobulins (mainly IgG) in intercellular substance of prickle-cell layer. In blood serum, circulating autoantibodies directed to intercellular substance.

Clues Acantholytic blisters, immunofluorescence pattern

Treatment Prednisone, 60 mg daily orally, and azothioprine, 150 mg daily. Greatly improved in 4 weeks. Maintenance: 12.5 mg prednisone and 100 mg azothioprine. Complications due to corticosteroid therapy: hyperglycemia (requiring insulin) and osteoporosis of vertebrae.

Bullous pemphigoid is a chronic bullous eruption in patients over 60 years of age and probably an autoimmune disorder.

EPIDEMIOLOGY

Age Sixty to eighty years or childhood
Sex Equal incidence in males and females

HISTORY

Duration of Lesions Often starts with a prodromal eruption (urticarial or eczematous lesions) and evolves in weeks to months to bullae which may appear suddenly as a generalized eruption
Skin Symptoms Usually none, except mouth lesions; occasionally moderate pruritus
Constitutional Symptoms None

PHYSICAL EXAMINATION

Skin Lesions

TYPE

Bullae, large, tense, firm-topped (Figure 41)
Erosions
Erythematous, urticarial-type lesions, not unlike the lesions in erythema multiforme

SHAPE Bullae are oval or round
ARRANGEMENT Arciform, annular, or serpiginous lesions are scattered and discrete

DISTRIBUTION Generalized or localized and randomly distributed
SITES OF PREDILECTION Axillae, medial aspect of thighs, groin, abdomen, flexor aspect of forearms
Mucous Membranes Mouth, anus, vagina: less severe and less painful than pemphigus (q.v.) and bullae less easily ruptured

DIFFERENTIAL DIAGNOSIS

Immunofluorescence usually permits a differentiation from pemphigus, erythema multiforme, or dermatitis herpetiformis.

DERMATOPATHOLOGY

Light Microscopy Subepidermal bullae, with regeneration of the floor of the bulla
Immunofluorescence Direct: IgG deposits along the basement membrane zone. Also C3, which may occur in the absence of IgG

TREATMENT

Systemic prednisone with starting doses of 50 to 100 mg to clear, combined with azathioprine for maintenance; or, preferably, azathioprine alone, 150 mg daily, for remission induction and 50 to 100 mg for maintenance

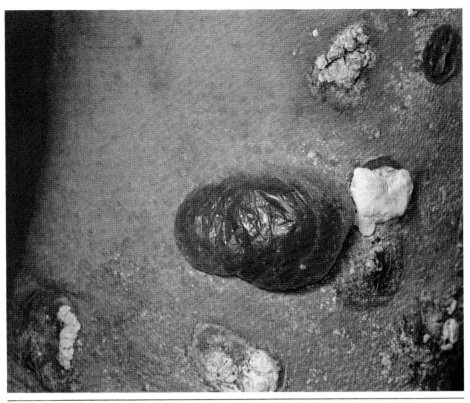

41 Bullous pemphigoid

Patient Profile Sixty-year-old female

History For 4 weeks, generalized, progressive bullous eruption. Mild diabetes, controlled by diet. No history of drugs; no other complaints.

Physical Examination Disseminated over the trunk and extremities, a large number of tense and flaccid bullae, varying in size from 1 to 4 cm. The adjacent skin is either normal or erythematous. Nikolsky's sign is negative. NOTE: White areas are remnants of ointment.

Differential Diagnosis Pemphigus vulgaris, bullous dermatitis herpetiformis, drug eruption, erythema multiforme

Laboratory and Special Examinations Histology: subepidermal bulla. Immunofluorescence: deposits of immunoglobulins and complement at the dermal-epidermal junction. In the blood serum, circulating autoantibodies directed to basement membrane.

Clues Flaccid bullae in older patients, gradual development (in contrast to pemphigus vulgaris), histology, immunofluorescence pattern

Treatment Oral azothioprine, 150 mg daily. After 4 weeks no new blisters and old ones healing. After 6 weeks all lesions healed. Maintenance: 100 mg azothioprine daily without difficulties.

Dermatitis Herpetiformis

This disease is a chronic, recurrent, intensely pruritic eruption occurring in *symmetrical* groups and comprised of three types of lesions: tiny vesicles, papules, and urticarial wheals.

EPIDEMIOLOGY

Age Twenty to sixty years, but most common at 30 to 40 years
Sex Male/female ratio 2:1

HISTORY

Duration of Lesions Days, weeks
Skin Symptoms Pruritus, intense, episodic; burning or stinging of the skin; pruritus may not occur

Systems Review Although laboratory evidence of small-bowel malabsorption occurs in 10 to 20 percent of patients, there are usually no symptoms.

PHYSICAL EXAMINATION
Skin Lesions

TYPE

Erythematous papule (Figure 42), tiny firm-topped vesicle sometimes

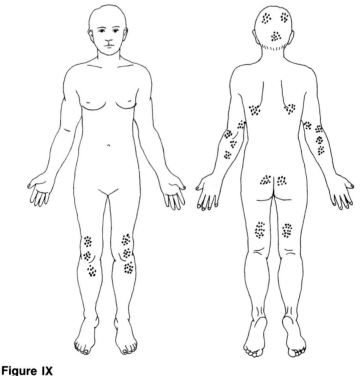

Figure IX
Dermatitis Herpetiformis

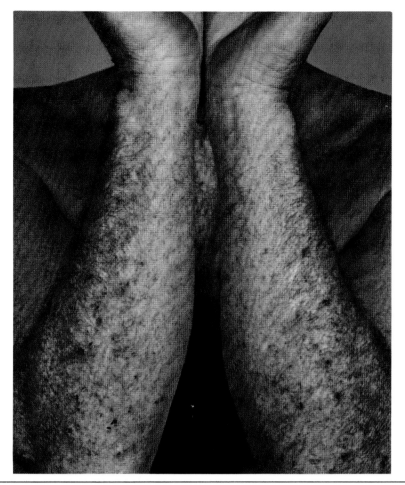

42 Dermatitis herpetiformis

Patient Profile *Fifty-eight-year-old male*

History *For 18 months, pruritic rash on arms and back. No other complaints. No use of drugs.*

Physical Examination *On the extensor surfaces of the forearms and in a horseshoe-shaped area on the lower back, disseminated, occasionally herpetiform, grouped, excoriated papules and a few small vesicles*

Differential Diagnosis *Scabies, eczema*

Laboratory and Special Examinations *Histology: dermal papillary collections of neutrophils, increased number of eosinophils, subepidermal vesicles containing some eosinophils. Immunofluorescence: granular deposits of IgA and C3 in dermal papillary tips. Small-intestinal biopsy: mild atrophy of villi and increased number of intraepithelial lymphocytes.*

Clues *Pruritic papules and vesicles on extensor surfaces of arms and lower back, histology, typical immunofluorescence pattern*

Treatment *Much improved under oral dapsone, 200 mg daily; later, maintenance with 50 mg daily. Gluten-free diet was not successful because of noncompliance of patient.*

hemorrhagic (Figure 43), or urticarial wheal
Occasionally bullae
Excoriations
Postinflammation spotty pigmentation

COLOR Red
SHAPE Round (all three types of lesions)
ARRANGEMENT In groups (hence the name *herpetiformis*)
DISTRIBUTION See Fig. IX. Regional (e.g., scalp) and symmetrical

SITES OF PREDILECTION

Extensor areas—elbows, knees
Buttocks, sacral area
Scalp, face, and hairline

DIFFERENTIAL DIAGNOSIS

Often difficut. Biopsy of early lesions is helpful, but immunofluorescence detecting IgA deposits in normal-appearing skin is the best confirmative evidence.

LABORATORY AND SPECIAL EXAMINATIONS

Dermatopathology Biopsy is best from early erythematous papule: (1) Microabscesses (polymorphonuclear cells and eosinophils) at the tips of the dermal papillae. Fibrin accumulation and necrosis occur also. (2) Dermal infiltration (severe) of neutrophils and eosinophils
Immunofluorescence (of Normal-appearing Skin, Usually the Buttocks) IgA deposits: (a) *linear,* band-like in the dermal papillae (other bullous diseases have, in addition, IgG in band-like pattern at the basement membrane zone); (b) *granular*—this correlates well with small-bowel disease.
Malabsorption Studies Steatorrhea (20 to 30 percent) and abnormal D-xylose absorption (10 to 73 percent)

Hematologic Anemia secondary to iron or folate deficiency

RADIOGRAPHIC STUDIES

Small bowel: In the proximal areas of the small intestine there is blunting and flattening of the villi (80 to 90 percent), as in celiac disease.

PATHOPHYSIOLOGY

The relationship of the gluten-sensitive enteropathy to the skin lesions has been controversial. It is now known that circulating immune complexes are always found in patients with dermatitis herpetiformis; these are probably deposited in the dermal papillae, causing the inflammatory process.

COURSE

Prolonged, for years, with a third of the patients eventually having a spontaneous remission

TREATMENT

Dapsone, 100 to 200 mg daily with gradual reduction to 25 to 50 mg. Obtain G-6-PD before starting treatment. Follow blood counts carefully.
Follow with weekly CBC for 1 month, then every 6 to 8 weeks.
If dapsone contraindicated or not tolerated, sulfapyridine 1.0 to 1.5 g daily, with plenty of fluids.
A gluten-free diet may completely suppress the disease or reduce the dosage of dapsone or sulfapyridine.

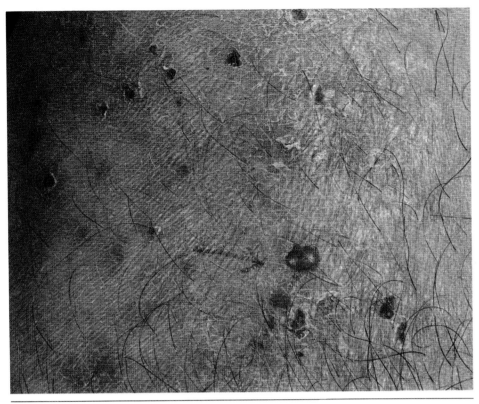

43   Dermatitis herpetiformis

Close-up view of excoriations and a few firm-topped vesicles (see Figure 42)

IX

Syndromes
Principally
Involving
Blood Vessels

Urticaria and Angioedema

Urticaria and angioedema are comprised of transient wheals (edematous papules and plaques, usually pruritic) and of larger edematous areas that involve the dermis and subcutaneous tissue (angioedema). Urticaria and/or angioedema may be acute or chronic recurrent. There are some syndromes with angioedema in which urticarial wheals are never present (e.g., hereditary angioedema).

ETIOLOGY

Angioedema and urticaria can be classified as IgE-mediated, hypocomplementemic, or related to physical stimuli (cold, sunlight, pressure), or idiosyncratic. A new syndrome, *angioedema-urticaria-eosinophilia syndrome,* is related to action of the eosinophil major basic protein.

Special Types

DERMOGRAPHIA Although 4.2% of the normal population have it, symptomatic dermographism is a nuisance problem. Fades in 30 min.

COLD URTICARIA Usually in children or young adults; "ice cube" test establishes diagnosis.

SOLAR URTICARIA Action spectra 290 to 500 nm, histamine is one of the mediators.

CHOLINERGIC URTICARIA Exercise to the point of sweating provokes typical lesions and establishes diagnosis.

HEREDITARY ANGIOEDEMA A serious autosomal dominant (positive family history) disorder; involves angioedema of face and extremities, episodes of laryngeal edema, and acute abdominal pain caused by angioedema of the bowel wall. Urticaria does not occur but there may be an erythema marginatum-like eruption. Laboratory abnormalities involve the complement system: decreased levels of C1 inactivator (85%) or dysfunctional inhibitor (15%), low C4 value in the presence of normal C1 and C3 levels. Angioedema results from bradykinin formation as C1 inactivator is also the major inhibitor of the Hageman factor and kallikrein, the two enzymes required for kinin formation.

VIBRATORY (PRESSURE) ANGIOEDEMA History of swelling induced by pressure (buttock swelling when seated, hand swelling after hammering, foot swelling after walking). No laboratory abnormalities; no fever. Antihistamines are ineffective but corticosteroids are sometimes helpful. Biopsy reveals a prominent mononuclear infiltrate in the deep dermis. Urticaria may occur in addition to angioedema. Vibratory angioedema may be familial (autosomal dominant) or sporadic. It is believed to result from histamine release from mast cells caused by "vibrating" stimuli—rubbing a towel across the back will produce lesions but direct pressure (without movement) will not cause a response.

ANGIOEDEMA-URTICARIA-EOSINOPHILIA SYNDROME Severe angioedema with pruritic urticaria involving the face, neck, extremities, and trunk that lasts for 7 to 10 days. There is fever and marked increase in normal weight (increased by 10 to 18%). No other organs are involved. Laboratory abnormalities include striking leukocytosis (20,000 to 70,000 per microliter) and eosinophilia (60 to 80% eosinophils) which are related to the severity of attack. There is an increase in IgM levels. There is no family history. Prognosis is good.

General Types

ACUTE URTICARIA (<30 DAYS) Often IgE-dependent with atopic background; antigens: food (milk, eggs, wheat, shellfish, nuts), therapeutic agents, drugs, cold, parasites, emotional stress (rare cause)

CHRONIC URTICARIA (>30 DAYS) Rarely IgE-dependent; ecology unknown in 80 to 90 percent; often emotional stress is an exacerbating factor

HISTORY

Duration of Lesions Hours

Skin Symptoms Pruritus, pain on walking (in foot involvement), flushing, burning, and wheezing (in cholinergic urticaria)

Constitutional Symptoms Fever in serum sickness and in the angioedema-urticaria-eosinophilia syndrome; in angioedema, hoarseness, stridor, dyspnea

Systems Review Arthralgia (serum sickness, necrotizing vasculitis, hepatitis)

PHYSICAL EXAMINATION

Skin Lesions

TYPE

Papules (wheals)—many, small (1 to 2 mm are typical in cholinergic urticaria), pruritic

Papules—small (1.0 cm) to large (8.0 cm), edematous plaques

Angioedema—skin-colored enlargement of portion of face (eyelids, lips, tongue) or extremity

COLOR   Pink with larger lesions having white central area surrounded by an erythematous halo

SHAPE   Oval, arciform, annular, polycyclic, serpiginous, and bizarre patterns

ARRANGEMENT   Annular, arciform, linear

DISTRIBUTION   Localized, regional, or generalized

SITES OF PREDILECTION   Sites of pressure, exposed areas (solar urticaria), trunk, hands and feet, lips, tongue, ears

DIAGNOSIS AND DIFFERENTIAL DIAGNOSIS

Wheals in urticaria usually disappear in 24 hours or much less, while persistent urticaria (> 96 hrs) is *necrotizing vasculitis,* and a biopsy should be done. *Cholinergic urticaria* can best be diagnosed by exercise to sweating. The *angioedema-urticaria-eosinophilia syndrome* has the following unusual features: fever, high leukocytosis (mostly eosinophils), striking increase in body weight, and a cyclic pattern that may occur and recur over a period of years.

LABORATORY AND SPECIAL EXAMINATIONS

For general medical work-up, to rule out systemic disease in chronic urticaria (systemic lupus erythematosus, necrotizing vasculitis, lymphoma)

Dermatopathology   Site: dermis. Edema of the dermis or subcutaneous tissue, dilation of venules, mast cell degranulation. In necrotizing vasculitis, biopsy is diagnostic. In angioedema-urticaria-eosinophilia syndrome, major basic protein is present outside the eosinophil around blood vessels and collagen bundles. There is dermal edema, a perivascular lymphocytic infiltration, and diffuse eosinophilic infiltration.

General Laboratory

SEROLOGIC   Search for hepatitis-associated antigen, assessment of the complement system, assessment of specific IgE antibodies by RAST in chronic urticaria

HEMATOLOGIC   The erythrocyte sedimentation rate is often elevated in urticaria perstans (necrotizing vasculitis); transient eosinophilia in urticaria from reactions to foods and drugs; high levels of eosinophilia in the angioedema-urticaria-eosinophilia syndrome.

Special Examination

Screening for functional C1 esterase inhibitor.

Ultrasonography for early diagnosis of bowel involvement; if abdominal pain is present this may indicate edema of the bowel.

PATHOPHYSIOLOGY

Lesions in acute urticaria result form antigen-induced release of biologically active materials from mast cells or basophilic leukocytes sensitized with specific IgE antibodies (Type I, anaphylactic hypersensitivity). Mediators released increase venular permeability, modulate the release of biologically active materials from other cell types. The angioedema-urticaria-eosinophilia syndrome may possibly result from the eosinophilia which is markedly elevated in the skin. In this syndrome the eosinophilia increases and decreases with the angioedema and urticaria; there are morphologic changes in the eosinophil including destruction and release of their contents in the dermis; major basic protein is distributed following release from the eosinophil into the collagen bundles, and mast cells in the dermis show degranulation.

COURSE AND PROGNOSIS

Half of the patients with urticaria alone are free of lesions in one year, but 20% have lesions for more than 20 years. Prognosis is good in most syndromes except hereditary angioedema, which may be fatal if untreated.

TREATMENT

Try to prevent attacks by elimination of etiologic chemicals or drugs: aspirin and food additives, especially in chronic recurrent urticaria—rarely successful

Antihistamines (H_1 blockers, e.g., hydroxyzine, terfenadine; and if they fail, H_1 and H_2 blockers, e.g., doxepin)

Prednisone is indicated for angioedema-urticaria-eosinophila syndrome

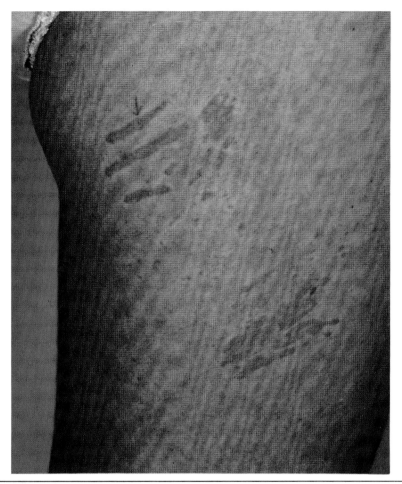

44 Urticaria

Patient Profile Seventeen-year-old female high school pupil

History For 3 months, daily eruptions of pruritic red spots

Physical Examination Chiefly on the outer side of the right leg, rose-red wheals, irregularly arranged, some of them linear. Moreover, linear wheals (arrow) provoked by firm stroking of the skin (dermographism).

Laboratory and Special Examinations Careful history for causative foods or drugs: negative. ESR and hematology: negative. Stool for helminthiasis: negative. Serologic for AST and ANA: negative.

Treatment Oral antihistamines. Gradual disappearance of the attacks.

This reaction pattern of blood vessels in the dermis with secondary epidermal changes is exhibited clinically as characteristic erythematous iris-shaped papules and vesicobullous lesions typically involving the extremities (especially the palms and soles) and the mucous membranes.

EPIDEMIOLOGY AND ETIOLOGY

Age Twenty to thirty years, with 50 percent under 20 years
Sex More males than females

Etiologies

DRUGS Sulfonamides, phenytoin, barbiturates, phenylbutazone, penicillin
INFECTION Especially following herpes simplex, *Mycoplasma*
IDIOPATHIC Fifty percent

HISTORY

Duration of Lesions Primary acute (hours) and recurrent acute episodes

Skin Symptoms None
Mucous Membrane Symptoms Mouth lesions are painful, tender
Constitutional Symptoms Fever, weakness, malaise

PHYSICAL EXAMINATION

Skin Lesions Lesions may develop over 10 days or more

TYPE

Macule —(48 hr)→ papule, 1 to 2 cm; lesions may appear for 2 weeks
Vesicles and bullae (in the center of the papule) (see Figure 45)

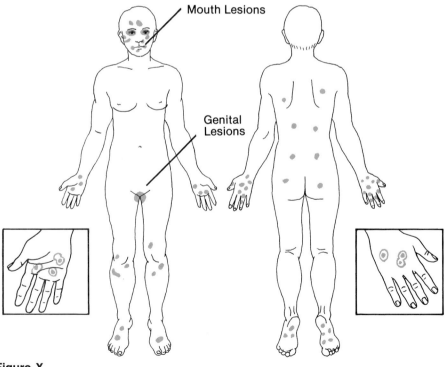

Mouth Lesions

Genital Lesions

Figure X
Erythema Multiforme

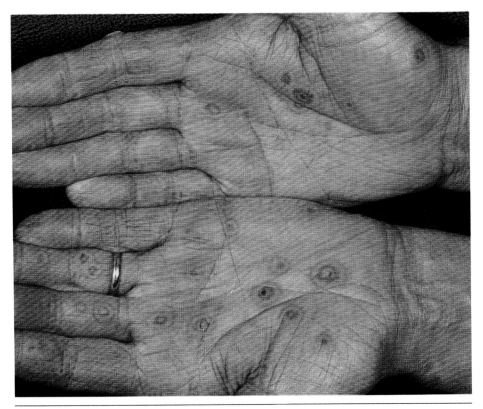

45 Erythema multiforme

Patient Profile Fifty-year-old female

History For 1 week, a rash on hands and arms. Not pruritic, no fever. No history of drugs. One year ago similar rash which cleared spontaneously in 3 weeks.

Physical Examination Symmetrically on the flexor sides of hands and forearms, edematous-looking, pale, erythematous-violaceous macules with a vesicle or an erosion in the center, surrounded by a few concentric rings, the outer ones being pale and the whole lesion resembling a "target."

Differential Diagnosis Urticaria

Laboratory and Special Examinations Histology: in the dermis a subepidermal vesicle, marked edema, and perivascular infiltrates consisting of polymorphonuclear leukocytes, histiocytes, lymphocytes, and a few eosinophils. Blood cell count and differential: no abnormalities.

Clues Typical "target" lesions, histology

Treatment Cleared spontaneously in 3 weeks

COLOR Dull red
SHAPE Iris or target lesions are typical
(see Figures 45 and 46)
ARRANGEMENT Localized to hands or
generalized
DISTRIBUTION Bilateral and often symmetrical
SITES OF PREDILECTION Dorsa of hands,
palms, and soles; forearms; feet; elbows
and knees; penis (50 percent) (see
Figure X)
Mucous Membrane Mouth and lips (99
percent)
Other Organs Pulmonary (30 percent),
eyes (91 percent) with corneal ulcers,
anterior uveitis

DIFFERENTIAL DIAGNOSIS

The target lesion and the symmetry are
quite typical and the diagnosis is not difficult. In the absence of skin lesions, the
mucous membrane lesions may present a
difficult differential diagnosis: bullous diseases and primary herpetic gingivostomatitis.

DERMATOPATHOLOGY

Site Epidermis and dermis
Process Inflammation characterized by
perivascular mononuclear infiltrate,
edema of the upper dermis; if bullae formation, there is eosinophilic necrosis of
keratinocytes with subepidermal bulla
formation

COURSE

Spontaneous remission in 2 to 3 weeks.
Recurrences are frequent (25 percent).

TREATMENT

Symptomatic. In severely ill patients,
systemic corticosteroids are usually
given (prednisone 50 to 80 mg daily
in divided doses, quickly tapered),
but their effectiveness has not been
established by controlled studies.
Control of herpes simplex using oral
acyclovir may prevent development
of the erythema multiforme syndrome.

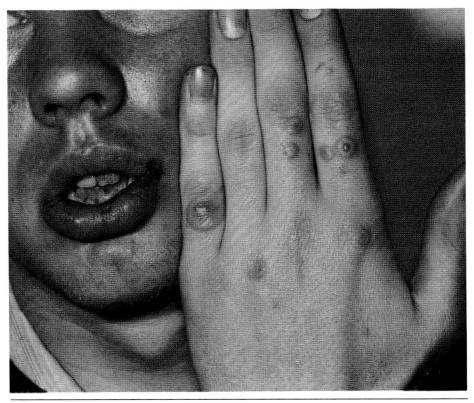

46 Erythema multiforme

Sixteen-year-old boy with typical target lesions on the hands, edema and erosions on the lower lip

Necrotizing Vasculitis Syndrome

This syndrome involves blood vessels (principally venules) with segmental inflammation and fibrinoid necrosis usually as a result of deposition of circulating immune complexes. Clinical manifestations include "palpable purpura" in the skin and vascular lesions chiefly in the kidney, muscles, joints, gastrointestinal tract, and peripheral nerves.

EPIDEMIOLOGY AND ETIOLOGY

Age All ages; in children known as Henoch-Schönlein purpura
Sex Equal incidence in males and females

Etiologies

IDIOPATHIC (50 percent)
DRUGS Sulfonamides, penicillin, serum
INFECTIONS Hepatitis B virus, group A hemolytic streptococcus, *Staphylococcus aureus, Mycobacterium leprae*
COLLAGEN VASCULAR DISEASE Systemic lupus erythematosus, rheumatoid arthritis, Sjögren syndrome
NEOPLASMS Lymphoproliferative disorders
MISCELLANEOUS Cryoglobulinemia, hypergammaglobulinemic purpura

HISTORY

Duration of Lesions Acute (days as in drug-induced or idiopathic), subacute (weeks, especially urticarial types), chronic (recurrent over years)
Skin Symptoms Pruritus, burning, pain, or no symptoms
Constitutional Symptoms Fever, malaise
Systems Review Symptoms of peripheral neuritis, abdominal pain, arthralgia, myalgia

PHYSICAL EXAMINATION

Skin Lesions

TYPE

"Palpable" purpura, petechiae (see Figure 47)
Urticarial wheals (persist more than 24 hr), (urticaria perstans)
Nodules, vesicles, necrotic ulcers

COLOR Purpuric lesions do not blanch (using a glass slide)
SHAPE Round, oval, annular, arciform

ARRANGEMENT Scattered, discrete lesions
DISTRIBUTION Usually regional localization: lower third of legs (Figure 47), ankles, buttocks (Figure 48), arms

DIFFERENTIAL DIAGNOSIS

An important differential is necrotizing vasculitis vs. *infarcts associated with bacteremia.* Biopsy may not be helpful in this differential. When faced with this dilemma in an acutely ill patient, antibiotic treatment is given, pending the result of the blood cultures. In the urticarial type the wheals are persistent (more than 24 hr), while all other types of urticarial wheals disappear completely in several hours.

LABORATORY AND SPECIAL EXAMINATIONS

Dermatopathology

SITE Dermis
PROCESS Desposition of fibrillary eosinophilic material (fibrinoid) in the walls of *venules* in the upper dermis, and perivenular inflammatory infiltrate (neutrophils in those patients with hypocomplementemia, and lymphocytes or neutrophils with normal serum complement). Extravasated red blood cells and fragmented neutrophils (nuclear "dust") are also present. C3 deposition is seen with immunofluorescence techniques. Perivenular IgA in Henoch-Schonlein syndrome.

General Laboratory Examinations

HEMATOLOGIC Increased erythrocyte sedimentation rate
SEROLOGIC Serum complement is reduced or normal in some patients, depending on associated disorders.
URINE Red cell casts, albuminuria

PATHOPHYSIOLOGY

The most frequently postulated mechanism for the production of necrotizing vasculitis is the deposition in tissues of

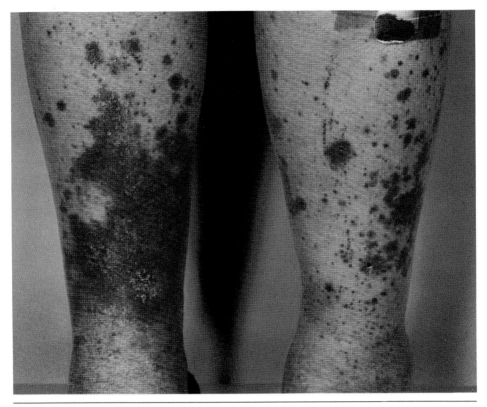

47   Necrotizing vasculitis

Patient Profile   Sixty-five-year-old female

History   For 6 weeks, rash on lower legs, not painful, not pruritic. Drugs: digoxin and a thiazide diuretic for 3 years

Physical Examination   On the lower legs, many red-violaceous, slightly indurated papules, varying in size from 0.5 to 5 cm, in part coalescing, particularly on the lower third of the legs. In general, the central parts of the spots are violaceous (purpura) which do not blanch with pressure (diascopy), while the peripheral parts are erythematous, blanching with pressure. Some central parts show, in addition, delicate hemorrhagic vesicles or erosions.

Laboratory and Special Examinations   BSR, hemoglobin, blood cell counts, and differential count: no abnormalities. Antistreptolysin titer: normal. ANA: negative. Circulating immune complexes in blood: increased. Urinalysis: normal. Histopathology: necrotizing vasculitis. Immunofluorescence of fresh lesions: deposits of immunoglobulins and complement in vessel walls.

Differential Diagnosis   Purpura due to bacteremias

Clues   Palpable purpura; besides purpura, erythematous areas, central vesiculation or necrosis, histology, immunofluorescence

Treatment   Temporary discontinuation of drugs did not influence the condition. Elastic bandages resulted in marked improvement. Spontaneous healing in 6 months.

circulating immune complexes. Initial alterations in venular permeability, which may facilitate the deposition of complexes at such sites, may be due to the release of vasoactive amines from platelets, basophils, and/or mast cells. Immune complexes may activate the complement system or may directly interact with Fc receptors on cell membranes. When the complement system is activated, the generation of anaphylatoxins C3a and C5a could degranulate mast cells. Also, C5a can attract neutrophils that could release lysosomal enzymes during phagocytosis of complexes and subsequently damage vascular tissue.

TREATMENT

Symptomatic. H_1 antihistamines, nonsteroidal anti-inflammatory agents, colchicine, dapsone, and rarely systemic corticosteroids.

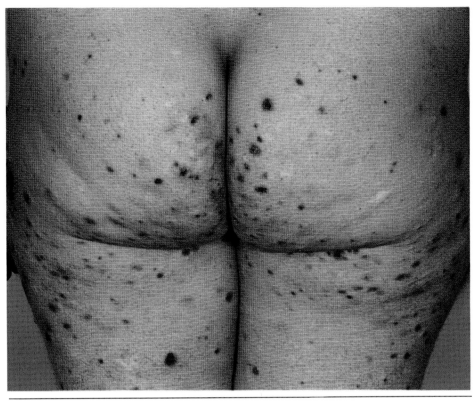

48 Necrotizing vasculitis

Female, aged 68, showing typical lesions on the lower legs, and also on the upper legs and buttocks. Some of the lesions show central necrosis.

Erythema nodosum is an important acute inflammatory/immunologic reaction pattern of the panniculus, characterized by the appearance of painful tender nodules on the lower legs and caused by multiple and diverse etiologies.

EPIDEMIOLOGY AND ETIOLOGY

Age Fifteen to thirty years, but age distribution related to etiology
Sex Three times more common in females than males

Etiologies

INFECTIOUS AGENTS Rarely primary tuberculosis (children), coccidioidomycosis, histoplasmosis, β-hemolytic streptococcus, *Yersinia* organisms, lymphogranuloma venereum
DRUGS Sulfonamides, oral contraceptives
MISCELLANEOUS Sarcoidosis, ulcerative colitis

HISTORY

Duration of Lesions Days
Skin Symptoms Painful, tender lesions
Constitutional Symptoms Fever, malaise
Systems Review Arthralgia (50 percent), other symptoms depending on etiology

PHYSICAL EXAMINATION

Skin Lesions

TYPE Nodules (3 to 20 cm) not sharply marginated (Figure 49)
COLOR Bright to deep red, later violaceous
PALPATION Indurated, tender
SHAPE Oval, round, arciform

ARRANGEMENT Scattered discrete lesions (2 to 50)
DISTRIBUTION Bilateral but not symmetrical
SITES OF PREDILECTION Lower legs (Figure 49), knees, arms, rarely face and neck

LABORATORY AND SPECIAL EXAMINATIONS

Radiologic examination of the chest is important to rule out sarcoidosis
Hepatitis antigens
ANA

DERMATOPATHOLOGY

Site Panniculus
Process Acute (polymorphonuclear) and chronic (granulomatous) inflammation in the panniculus and around blood vessels in the septum and adjacent fat

COURSE

Spontaneous resolution occurs in 6 weeks but the course depends on the etiology.

TREATMENT

Bed rest. Symptomatic anti-inflammatory treatment: salicylates, iodides. The use of systemic corticosteroids is indicated only when the etiology is known.

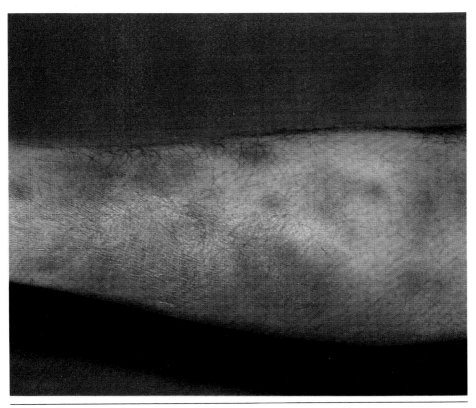

49 Erythema nodosum

Patient Profile   Thirty-seven-year-old male

History   For 3 weeks, painful red lesions on lower legs. No fever. Had no complaints previously. No history of drugs.

Physical Examination   On the sides and front of lower legs, red, warm, in part nodular, indurated lesions 2 to 5 cm in size, often merging to larger lesions. The borders are not well-defined.

Differential Diagnosis   Superficial thrombophlebitis, nonspecific panniculitis, erysipelas

Laboratory and Special Examinations   BSR = 40, blood cell count, and differential: normal. AST: 100 U. Serologic tests for syphilis and rheumatoid arthritis: negative. BUN, creatinine, alkaline phosphate: normal. Chest x-ray; normal. Culture of sputum and trachea negative for tuberculosis and streptococci. Tests for Yersinia: negative. Histology: perivascular infiltrates, mainly lymphocytes and histiocytes and a few polymorphonuclear leukocytes. Some necrosis of fat cells. Conclusion: nonspecific panniculitis. Immunofluorescence: negative.

Clues   Multiple, warm, painful nodular infiltrates on lower legs; histology. In this case the cause remained unknown, which is not rare.

Treatment   None. Spontaneous resolution in 6 weeks.

X

Lupus

Erythematosus

Systemic Lupus Erythematosus (SLE)

This serious multisystem disease involves connective tissue and blood vessels; the clinical manifestations include fever (90 percent); skin lesions (85 percent); arthritis; and renal, cardiac, and pulmonary disease. Systemic lupus erythematosus may uncommonly develop in patients with chronic discoid lupus erythematosus (DLE).

EPIDEMIOLOGY AND ETIOLOGY

Age Thirty (females), 40 (males)
Sex Male/female ratio 1:8
Race More common in blacks
Other Features Family history (less than 5 percent); SLE syndrome can be induced by drugs (hydralazine, certain anticonvulsants, and procainamide), although rash is an uncommon feature of drug-induced SLE. Sunlight may cause an exacerbation of SLE (36 percent).

HISTORY

Duration of Lesions Weeks (acute), months
Skin Symptoms Pruritus (especially papular lesions)
Constitutional Symptoms Fatigue (100 percent), fever (100 percent), weight loss, and malaise
Systems Review Arthralgia or arthritis, abdominal pain

PHYSICAL EXAMINATION

Skin Lesions

TYPE

Erythematous, confluent, macular butterfly eruption (face) with fine scaling (Figure 51)
Erythematous, discrete, papular or urticarial lesions (face and arms)
Bullae, often hemorrhagic (acute flares)
Discoid plaques as in chronic discoid lupus erythematosus (face and arms) (see Figure 51)
"Palpable" purpura (vasculitis)

COLOR Bright red (see Figures 50 and 51)
SHAPE Round or oval

ARRANGEMENT

Diffuse involvement of the face in light-exposed areas
Scattered discrete lesions (face, forearms, and dorsa of hands)

DISTRIBUTION Localized or generalized
SITES OF PREDILECTION Face (80 percent); scalp (discoid lesions); dorsa of the forearms, hands, fingers, fingertips (vasculitis); palms; periungual telangiectases and palmar erythema are also seen

Hair

Discoid lesions associated with patchy alopecia
Diffuse alopecia

Mucous Membranes Ulcers arising in purpuric necrotic lesions on palate (80 percent), buccal mucosa, or gums
Extracutaneous Multisystem Involvement Arthralgia or arthritis (15 percent), renal disease (50 percent), pericarditis (20 percent), pneumonitis (20 percent), gastrointestinal (due to arteritis and sterile peritonitis), hepatomegaly (30 percent), splenomegaly (20 percent), lymphadenopathy (50 percent), peripheral neuropathy (14 percent), central nervous system disease (10 percent), seizures or organic brain disease (14 percent)

DERMATOPATHOLOGY

Skin Atrophy of epidermis, liquefaction degeneration of the dermal-epidermal junction, edema of the dermis, dermal inflammatory infiltrate (lymphocytes), and fibrinoid degeneration of the connective tissue and walls of the blood vessels
Other Organs The fundamental lesion is fibrinoid degeneration of connective tissue and walls of the blood vessels, which is associated with an inflammatory infiltrate of plasma cells and lymphocytes.
Immunofluorescence of Skin The "lupus band test" (a direct fluorescence antibody test measuring IgG, IgM, and C1q) shows a granular or globular pattern along the dermal-epidermal junction. This is positive in the lesional skin

in 90 percent and in clinically normal skin (sun-exposed, 70 to 80 percent; non-sun-exposed, 50 percent)

LABORATORY AND SPECIAL EXAMINATIONS

Serologic   ANA positive ($>$95 percent), peripheral pattern of nuclear fluorescence is very specific for SLE, low levels of complement (especially with renal involvement). SS-A(Ro) autoantibodies are present in a subset of subacute cutaneous lupus erythematosus (SCLE) in which there is skin involvement and photosensitivity. SS-B(La) antibodies also coexist in 50 percent of the cases.

Hematologic   Anemia [normocytic, normochromic, or rarely hemolytic Coombs positive, leukopenia (less than $4000/mm^3$)], elevated erythrocyte sedimentation rate (a good guide to activity of the disease)

PATHOPHYSIOLOGY

The tissue injury in the epidermis results from the deposition of immune complexes at the dermal-epidermal junction. Immune complexes selectively generate the assembly of the membrane-attack complex, which mediates membrane injury.

TREATMENT

General measures: rest, avoidance of sun exposure.

Indications for prednisone (60 mg daily in divided doses): (1) CNS involvement, (2) renal involvement, (3) severely ill patients without CNS (4) hemolytic crisis.

Chloroquine sulfate or other antimalarials are useful for treatment of the skin lesions but do not reduce the need for prednisone. See precautions in the use of chloroquine on page 138.

PROGNOSIS

Five-year survival is 93 percent.

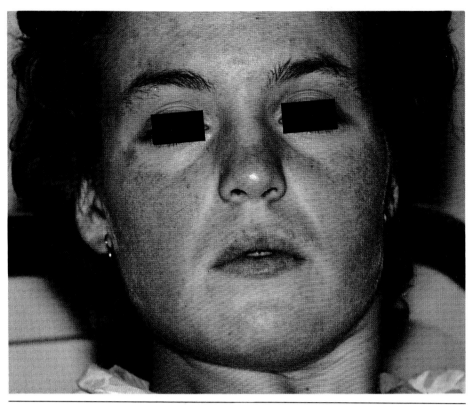

50 Systemic lupus erythematosus

Patient Profile *Twenty-year-old female*

History *For 4 weeks, a rash on the face and progressive malaise. For 1 week, fever (39°C), painful joints on motion, and photosensitivity.*

Physical Examination *On the face, an erythematous, very slightly edematous, sharply outlined blush in the "butterfly area." A few erythematous, slightly indurated spots on the fingers. Acrocyanosis and Raynaud's phenomenon.*

Differential Diagnosis *Photodermatosis (e.g., due to drugs), rosacea, seborrheic dermatitis*

Laboratory and Special Examinations *Blood: BSR = 100 mm, anemia, leukopenia (WBC = 3000/mm³), false-positive STS, TPI and Reiter negative, positive tests for rheumatoid arthritis, ANA positive, LE cells strongly positive, decreased total serum complement level. Urinalysis: proteinuria. Histopathology: some atrophy of epidermis, liquefaction degeneration of basal layer, edema in upper dermis, infiltrates of lymphocytes scattered through dermis around vessels. Immunofluorescence (lesion and noninvolved skin): granular deposits of IgG at dermal-epidermal junction.*

Clues *Blush in butterfly area, internal and laboratory manifestations, histology, immunofluorescence of normal and involved skin*

Chronic Discoid Lupus Erythematosus (CDLE)

This chronic, indolent skin disease is characterized by sharply marginated, scaly, atrophic, red plaques, usually occurring on the habitually exposed areas.

EPIDEMIOLOGY

Age Twenty to forty-five years
Sex Females
Race Possibly more severe in blacks

HISTORY

Duration of Lesions Months
Skin Symptoms Usually none, sometimes slightly pruritic
Systems Review Negative

PHYSICAL EXAMINATION
Skin Lesions

TYPE

Early Papules and plaques, sharply marginated, with slight adherent scaling
Later Atrophy and depression of lesions, with slightly raised border (Figure 51). Erythema is comprised of fine telangiectases (Figure 50). Follicular plugging (closely set and often in clusters)
COLOR Active lesions bright red. "Burned out" may be pink scars or white (hypomelanosis) macules. Lesions may show hyperpigmentation, especially in the ear.
SHAPE Round, oval, annular, polycyclic with irregular borders
DISTRIBUTION Scattered discrete lesions
SITES OF PREDILECTION Face, scalp, nose, dorsa of forearms, hands, fingers, toes, and less frequently the trunk
Hair Alopecia associated with lesions in the scalp skin
Mucous Membranes Less than 5 percent of patients have lip involvement (hyperkeratosis and erythema) and atrophic erythematous areas with or without ulceration on the buccal mucosa, tongue, and palate

DIFFERENTIAL DIAGNOSIS

The lesions of discoid lupus erythematosus may closely mimic *actinic keratosis.* *Plaque psoriasis* and scaling discoid lupus erythematosus may be virtually indistinguishable, especially on the dorsa of the hands. (The histopathology of discoid lupus erythematosus permits distinction of the two.) Polymorphous light eruption (PMLE) may pose a problem. (PMLE dis-appears in the winter in northern latitudes; PMLE does not develop atrophy or follicular plugging; PMLE does not occur in unexposed areas—mouth, hairy scalp.)

LABORATORY AND SPECIAL EXAMINATIONS

Dermatopathology The typical lesions show a classic picture: hyperkeratosis, atrophy of the epidermis, follicular plugging, liquefaction degeneration of the basal cell layer. In the dermis there is edema, dilation of small blood vessels, and perifollicular and periappendageal inflammatory infiltrate (lymphocytes and histiocytes). Strong PAS reaction staining of the subepidermal, thickened basement zone.
Immunofluorescence Positive in active lesions at least 6 weeks old. Granular deposits of IgG at the dermal-epidermal junction. This is known as the *lupus band test* (LBT) and is positive in 90 percent of the lesions but *negative in the normal skin* (both sun-exposed and nonexposed), while systemic lupus erythematosus (SLE) has a positive LBT in lesional as well as both normal sun-exposed (70 to 80 percent) and nonexposed (50 percent) skin.

General Laboratory Examination

SEROLOGIC Low incidence of ANA in a titer more than 1:16
HEMATOLOGIC Occasionally a leukopenia (less than 4500/mm^3)

COURSE AND PROGNOSIS

Only 1 to 5 percent may develop SLE; complete remission occurs in 40 percent.

TREATMENT

Topical sunscreens (SPF 15) routinely
Topical fluorinated corticosteroids (with caution)
Intralesional triamcinolone acetonide, 5 mg/ml, for small lesions
Chloroquine sulfate, 250 mg bid or hydroxychloroquine, 400 mg bid
Pretreatment eye examinations are important as chloroquine retinopathy has been reported.

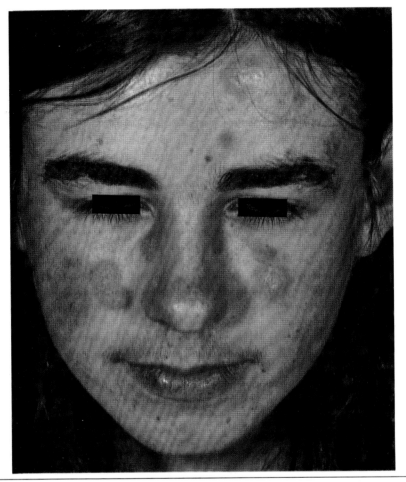

51 Chronic discoid lupus erythematosus

Patient Profile Seventeen-year-old Caucasian female

History For 3 months, red lesions on the face, occasionally pruritic. No other complaints. Did not respond to betamethasone-17-valerate cream. Worse on sun exposure.

Physical Examination Round to ovoid, slightly indurated, red-violaceous patches, fairly sharply demarcated, disseminated on the face, predominantly in the "butterfly" area. Most patches show a slight follicular keratotic scaling, and some show central atrophy. Similar lesions on the left lower arm, and on the light-exposed area of the upper chest. General physical examination: no abnormalities.

Differential Diagnosis Systemic lupus erythematosus, rosacea, psoriasis, tinea

Laboratory and Special Examinations Histology: atrophy of epidermis, follicular hyperkeratosis, vacuolization of basal cells, slight perivascular round-cell infiltrates in upper dermis. Immunofluorescence: IgG deposits along dermal-epidermal junction. Noninvolved skin: negative. ESR, hemoglobin, white blood cell count, and urinalysis: normal. ANA: low-grade positive. LE cell phenomenon: negative.

Clues Indurated, keratotic and atrophic patches; site; histology; immunofluorescence

Treatment Much improved under corticosteroid creams with plastic occlusion and intralesional corticosteroids. In summertime: sunscreens.

XI

Metabolic

and Heritable

Disorders

Porphyria
Xanthomas
Vitiligo
Neurofibromatosis
Ichthyosis

Porphyria Cutanea Tarda

This metabolic disease is expressed clinically as vesicles and bullae with scarring, largely in light-exposed areas subject to repeated trauma, i.e., the dorsa of the hands. Porphyria cutanea tarda (PCT) is usually induced by drugs or chemicals, but may be hereditary.

EPIDEMIOLOGY AND ETIOLOGY

Age Thirty to forty, rarely in children
Sex Males more than females
Heredity Possibly autosomal dominant in some patients
Chemicals and Drugs that Induce PCT Ethanol, estrogens, and chloroquine provoke PCT in genetically susceptible persons, while hexachlorobenzene and chlorinated phenols affect normal persons.
Other Factors Diabetes mellitus in 25 percent; rarely hepatoma

HISTORY

Duration of Lesions Gradual (weeks) during repeated exposures to sunlight
Symptoms Patient does not present with photosensitivity but complains of "fragile skin" that forms blisters.
Systems Review Negative, unlike porphyria variegata (see Differential Diagnosis). Acute attacks are absent.

PHYSICAL EXAMINATION

Skin Lesions

TYPE

Vesicles or bullae—round, oval, or linear; tense; firm roof (see Figure 52)
Erosions
Pink atrophic scars at sites of previous bullae (see Figure 52)
Milia, 1.0 to 2.0 mm, (see Figure 52) on dorsa of hands
"Heliotrope" (violaceous suffusion) in the periorbital skin
Hypertrichosis (may be presenting feature) on the face
Sclerodermoid, diffuse involvement: on the exposed areas, especially face and chest

DISTRIBUTION Dorsa of hands and feet (toes), nose, upper trunk (see Figure XI)

DIFFERENTIAL DIAGNOSIS

"Pseudo-PCT": Drugs (sulfonamides, nalidixic acid, furosemide, naproxen, tetracycline), hemodialysis, epidermolysis bullosa acquisita, which has the clinical picture (increased skin fragility, easy bruising, and light-provoked bullae), the histology (subepidermal bullae with little or no dermal inflammation, and thickened dermal capillary walls with deposition of periodic acid-Schiff positive material), and the findings of immunofluorescent studies (IgG and C, deposition around vessels, and patchy, granular immunoglobulin deposition at the dermal-epidermal junction) combine to form a distinctive syndrome, and only the absence of the defect in porphyrin metabolism prevents a firm diagnosis of porphyria cutanea tarda.
Porphyria variegata (PV), an autosomal dominant, potentially fatal disease following ingestion of barbiturates and sulfonamides, has identical skin lesions to PCT. High stool protoporphyrin is distinctive for PV. Also PV patients have acute attacks, usually precipitated by drugs and characterized by acute abdominal pain, and elevated levels of porphobilinogen can be detected in the urine by the Watson-Schwartz test.

LABORATORY EXAMINATIONS

Blood Chemistry Increased serum iron (66 percent), increased iron storage in the liver, diabetes mellitus (25 percent)
Porphyrin Studies

IN URINE Increased uroporphyrin (type I > III) and 7-carboxyl porphyrins (III > I)
IN FECES Increased isocoproporphyrin
Wood's Lamp Pink fluorescence of the urine; add 5 ml of 5% hydrochloric acid to increase fluorescence

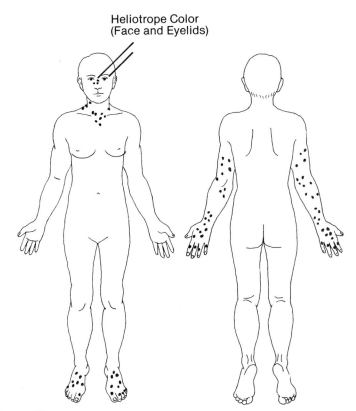

Heliotrope Color
(Face and Eyelids)

Figure XI
Porphyria Cutanea Tarda

PATHOPHYSIOLOGY

All porphyrias except PCT are known to result from a specific enzymatic defect in the heme biosynthetic pathway. The inherited nature of a specific enzymatic defect has not been established in PCT. It is now known, however, that there is a reduced activity of hepatic uroporphyrinogen decarboxylase, which is specific for patients with PCT. This enzymatic defect is intrinsic and not acquired and is present in hepatic cells and, in some patients, also in the erythrocytes. The cause of the hepatic siderosis in PCT is not known.

TREATMENT

Stop ethanol or estrogens or other chemicals.

Phlebotomy is the treatment of choice—500 ml weekly or biweekly until hemoglobin is 10 to 11 g/100 ml or until serum iron is reduced to 50 to 60 μg/100 ml. Clinical remission occurs after 6 to 9 months, and biochemical remission may require 12 to 24 months. Remissions of 1 to 8 years occur with phlebotomy.

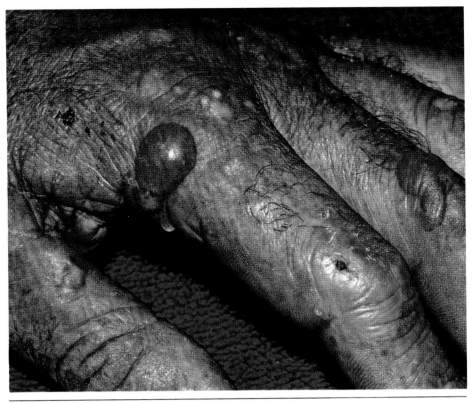

52 Porphyria cutanea tarda

Patient Profile *Fifty-five-year-old gardener*

History *For 3 months, blistering on hands following slight mechanical injuries, possibly worse on sunny days. Moderate alcohol intake, no drugs, family history not contributory, no other complaints.*

Physical Examination *On extensor surface of both hands, predominantly on the fingers, are three blisters, filled with clear fluid. Elsewhere are remnants of blisters, and on the second metacarpophalangeal joint are two small white papules of hard consistency (milia).*

Laboratory and Special Examinations *Urine: orange-red fluorescence under Wood's light (after a few drops of acid had been added), strongly elevated excretion of uroporphyrin I (460 μg per 24 hr; upper normal limit 100 μg). Feces: marked elevation of uro- and coproporphyrin, normal precursors. Blood: increased serum iron level. Histopathology: subepidermal blister.*

Clues *Blistering on extensor sides of hands, milia, elevated urinary and fecal porphyrin excretion, elevated serum iron*

Treatment *Series of phlebotomies for 6 months gave almost complete relief of symptoms. Discontinuation of alcohol intake.*

Erythropoietic Protoporphyria (EPP)

This hereditary metabolic disease is manifested, often in early childhood, as an acute photosensitivity resembling an exaggerated sunburn: erythema, edema, blisters.

EPIDEMIOLOGY AND ETIOLOGY

Age One to four years, mild cases may not be discovered until adulthood
Heredity Autosomal dominant

HISTORY

Duration of Onset of Lesions Immediate (minutes) after sunlight exposure (even through window glass)
Skin Symptoms In sequence: stinging, burning, pruritus, swelling
Systems Review Biliary colic, even in children, cholelithiasis (rare)

PHYSICAL EXAMINATION
Skin Lesions

EARLY STAGES

"Sunburn": erythema, edema—confluent, *no rash*
Rare bullae (especially on the nose), erosions, crusts
Purpura (especially on the nose and hands)
Urticaria (rare)

LATE STAGES

Scars—atrophic, waxy
"Aged knuckles"—thickened, waxy, wrinkled over dorsa of hands
Diffuse infiltration and wrinkling of the face (see Figure 53)

DISTRIBUTION Face (see Figure 53): nose, cheeks, periorbital, ears; dorsa of hands

DIFFERENTIAL DIAGNOSIS

Exaggerated sunburn (not a rash) following short exposures, with immediate stinging and burning, is a rare presentation in any kind of photosensitivity except EPP.

LABORATORY EXAMINATIONS
Porphyrin Studies

Red blood cells and stool: increased protoporphyrin
Urine has no change in level of porphyrins
Decreased activity of ferrochelatase in bone marrow, liver, and skin fibroblasts
Blood Demonstration of fluorescence in red blood cells establishes diagnosis—easily done and immediate results

RADIOGRAPHY

Gallstones may be present (uncommon).

TREATMENT

Beta-carotene capsules (Solatene, Roche), 90 to 180 mg daily to achieve levels of 600 to 800 μg per 100 ml. Therapeutic effect may be delayed for 1 to 2 months.
Patients with EPP have severely restricted lives. Treatment with beta-carotene will improve their sun tolerance by a few hours and improve their lifestyle. Long exposure, however, is never achieved.
Oral PUVA phototherapy has recently been shown to improve sun tolerance when combined with beta carotene.

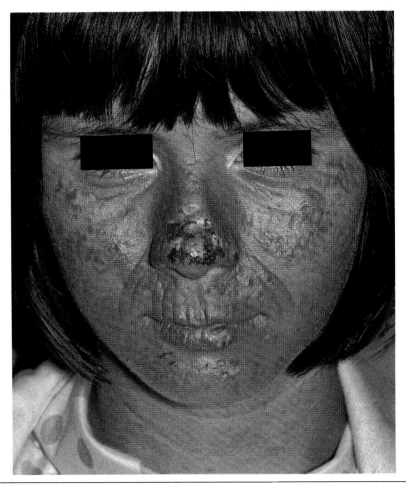

53 Erythropoietic protoporphyria

Patient Profile   Fifteen-year-old Caucasian girl

History   Since first year of life, severe sensitivity to sunlight. After 5-min exposure to sunlight, stinging and burning sensations followed a few hours later by redness and swelling; occasionally also erosive and crusted lesions which heal in 1 or 2 weeks. A younger sister has similar complaints. Topical sunscreens gave no relief.

Physical Examination   The nose, lower lip, and chin show erythematous, in part erosive and crusted, lesions. On both cheeks, erythematous lesions. Nose and cheeks in addition show a few small slightly depressed scars and peculiar waxy thickening of skin. Linear scars are present between the nose and mouth.

Differential Diagnosis   Congenital porphyria of Günther, lipoid proteinosis

Laboratory and Special Examinations   Blood: 10 percent of the erythrocytes show spontaneous red fluorescence when examined under a fluorescence microscope. Red blood cell protoporphyrin: 900 μg per 100 ml of cells (upper normal limit: 150); plasma protoporphyrin: 30 (normal: trace); fecal protoporphyrin: 185 (normal: 50). Urine: no excess of porphyrins.

Clues   Sunlight sensitivity, onset in early childhood, familial occurrence, delicate scarring, fluorescing erythrocytes, elevated protoporphyrin levels in blood

Treatment   Beta-carotene orally, 175 mg daily during the summer with poor response

Xanthomas

GENERAL REMARKS

Cutaneous xanthomas are yellow-brown, pinkish, or orange macules (xanthoma striatum), papules (xanthoma eruptivum), plaques (xanthelasma palpebrarum), nodules (xanthoma tuberosum), or infiltrations in tendons (xanthoma tendinosum). Xanthomas are characterized by accumulations of xanthoma cells—macrophages containing droplets of lipids. A xanthoma may be a symptom of a general metabolic disease, a generalized histiocytosis, or a local cell dysfunction. The following classification is based on this principle: (1) xanthomas due to hyperlipoproteinemia (hyperlipidemia) and (2) normolipoproteinemic xanthomas. Of the latter group only the normolipoproteinemic xanthelasmata of the eyelids are common enough to be discussed in this book. Although the hyperlipoproteinemic xanthomas are relatively rare, they are important for two reasons: (1) They may be the first symptom of a serious metabolic disease. (2) They may be regarded as an experiment of nature which may enable us to study the pathogenesis of atherosclerotic disease.

The causes of hyperlipoproteinemic xanthomas may be divided into primary, in most cases genetically determined, and secondary, those caused by severe hypothyroidism, biliary cirrhosis, and a number of still rarer conditions. Those hyperlipoproteinemias that are related to diabetes may be divided into those associated with insulin-dependent diabetes or with maturity-onset diabetes.

Fredrickson pointed out in his classification that hypercholesterolemia, hypertriglyceridemia, and hyperphospholipidemia are caused by elevation of one or more of the four classes of lipoproteins, which are carriers of the lipids. Each class carries lipids in a different proportion. The high-density lipoproteins (HDL) carry the highest proportion of proteins and phospholipids; the low-density lipoproteins (LDL) carry the highest proportion of cholesterol and its esters; the very low density lipoproteins (VLDL) carry a high proportion of triglycerides; the chylomicrons carry almost only triglycerides. This explains why a hypercholesterolemia may as well be caused by an elevated LDL as by an elevated VLDL level. A hypercholesterolemia due to VLDL is necessarily accompanied (contrary to one caused by elevated LDL) by hypertriglyceridemia. It is important to recognize this because the pathologic consequences of elevated LDL are much more serious than those caused by elevated VLDL. With minor changes and expansions the concept of Fredrickson is still accepted (see Table A).

Table B summarizes the features of the hyperlipoproteinemias.

GENETIC ASPECTS

Familial hypercholesterolemia is a dominant hereditary disease with the phenotype II[a]. In its heterozygous form it is very often complicated by atherosclerotic cardiovascular disease (ASCVD). The homozygous form is always accompanied by extremely high lipid levels and severe ASCVD, generally lethal before 20 years of age. Familial hypercholesterolemia is due to a hereditary defect in the LDL receptor on the cells. The best therapeutic results may be expected from a diet low in cholesterol combined with bile acid sequestrants (cholestramine) and HMG CoA reductase inhibitors. It is resistant to a low-cholesterol diet, cholestyramine, and nicotinic acid derivatives. In homozygous patients, portocaval shunt must be considered. Promising is therapy with HMG CoA reductase inhibitors, which are still under investigation.

Combined hypercholesterolemia is a genetically heterogeneous disease manifesting itself as types II[a], II[b], and IV.

Polano MK et al: *Arch Dermatol* **100**:387—400, 1969
Vermeer BJ et al: *Br J Dermatol* **100**:657—666, 1979

Table A Common Abnormal Lipoprotein Patterns in Hyperlipoproteinemia

Type	Lipoprotein abnormalities	Appearance of plasma*	Usual changes in lipid concentrations
I	Massive chylomicronemia VLDL, LDL, HDL normal or decreased	Cream layer on top, clear below	C ↑, TG ↑ ↑
IIᵃ	LDL increased VLDL normal	Clear	C ↑, TG normal
IIᵇ	LDL increased VLDL increased	May be slightly turbid	C ↑, TG ↑
III	Presence of β-VLDL	Usually turbid, often with faint cream layer	C ↑, TG ↑ ↑
IV	VLDL increased	Usually turbid, no cream layer	C normal, TG ↑ ↑
V	Chylomicrons present VLDL increased	Cream layer on top, turbid below	C ↑, TG ↑ ↑

*After standing at 4°C for 18 hr or more.

NOTE   VLDL = very low density (alpha) lipoproteins; LDL = low density (beta) lipoproteins; HDL = high density (alpha) lipoproteins; C = cholesterol; TG = triglycerides; β-VLDL = IDL = intermediate density lipoproteins.

Source   Modified from Frederickson DS: Plasma lipid abnormalities and cutaneous and subcutaneous xanthomas, in *Dermatology in General Medicine*. Edited by TB Fitzpatrick et al. McGraw–Hill, New York, 1979, p. 1120.

Table B   Classification of Xanthomas

Xanthelasma palpebrarum	Normolipemic or types IIᵃ, IIᵇ, III
Xanthoma tendineum	Types IIᵃ, IIᵇ, III
Xanthoma tuberosum	Types IIᵃ, IIᵇ, III
Xanthoma papuloeruptivum	Types I, III, IV/V
Xanthoma chromia and xanthoma striatum palmare	Type III

Type III, although familial, is not clearly characterized genetically. Typical are the yellow streaks in the palms, which may be at the skin level or elevated. Association with ASCVD and atherosclerosis of peripheral vessels is reported. The xanthomata usually precede the ASCVD. The patients react favorably to a low-carbohydrate, low-caloric diet.

Types IV/V may be familial without a distinct hereditary pattern; generally an abnormal glucose tolerance is present. There is not an increased incidence of ASCVD. The papuloeruptive xanthomas are more widely disseminated on the trunk and feet than in type III. There is a good response to a low-carbohydrate, low-caloric diet and abstinence from alcohol.

Xanthelasma Palpebrarum (Eyelid Xanthoma)

Xanthelasma palpebrarum *may* or *may not* be associated with hyperlipoproteinemia. When hyperlipoproteinemia is present this may be of type II^a, II^b, or III.

EPIDEMIOLOGY AND ETIOLOGY

Age Fifty years; children or young adults if associated with type II or III pattern
Sex Either
Incidence Most common of all xanthomas
Significance May be an isolated finding unrelated to hyperlipoproteinemia, but sometimes there is elevation of LDL. When the LDL is markedly elevated, it is a sign of hyperlipoproteinemia.

HISTORY

Duration of Lesions Months, with slow enlargement from tiny spot
Skin Symptoms None

PHYSICAL EXAMINATION

Skin Lesions

TYPE   Plaques, soft
COLOR   Yellow-orange
SHAPE   Polygonal
DISTRIBUTION   Localized to eyelids

DIFFERENTIAL DIAGNOSIS

Quite typical but early lesions can be confused with milia, and biopsy is necessary in small lesions.

LABORATORY EXAMINATION

Cholesterol estimation in plasma, if enhanced screening for type of hyperlipoproteinemia

PROGNOSIS

If due to hyperlipoproteinemia, complication with ASCVD may be expected.

TREATMENT

Excision or applications of trichloroacetic acid are the treatments of choice; however, recurrences are not uncommon.

SIGNIFICANCE

In a larger proportion of the patients with xanthelasmata palpebralia no metabolic disturbances are found. In others, xanthelasmata palpebralia are a sign of familial hyperlipoproteinemia types II^a, II^b, or III. When total lipids and total cholesterol content of the serum are within normal limits, no further lipid analysis is necessary.

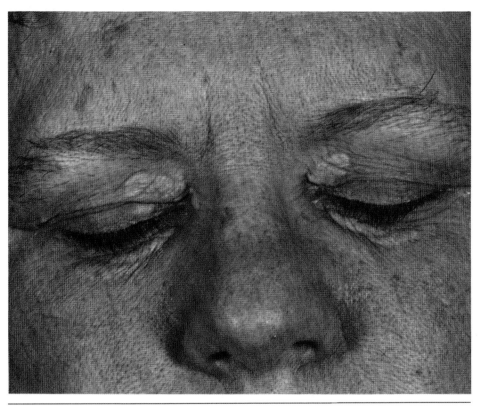

54 Xanthelasmata palpebralia (normolipemic)

Patient Profile Sixty-nine-year-old female

History For 5 years, yellow spots around the eyes

Physical Examination On the nasal part of inferior and superior eyelids, longitudinal, yellow-brown, slightly elevated infiltrations 1.0 to 2.5 cm in length and 0.5 to 0.7 cm in width. Otherwise no xanthomata.

Differential Diagnosis Xanthelasmata palpebralia with or without hyperlipoproteinemia

Blood Chemistry Total lipids 838 mg per 100 ml. Total cholesterol 230 mg per 100 ml. (normal)

Clues Clinical picture, blood chemistry

Treatment After three applications of trichloroacetic acid the lesions cleared. Recurrences after 2 years, reacted again with this treatment.

Xanthoma Tendinum

In xanthoma tendinum, yellow subcutaneous infiltrates move together with the extensor tendons. It is associated with type II^a, II^b, and III patterns.

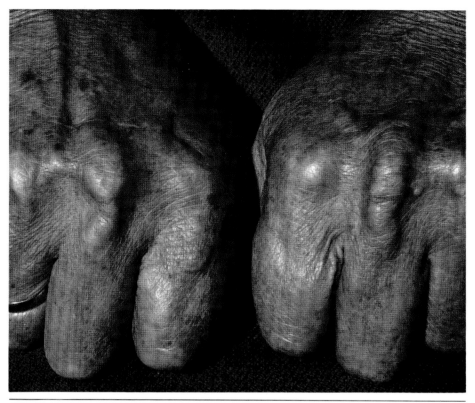

55 Xanthomata tendinea in hyperlipoproteinemia, type II[a]

Patient Profile   Fifty-four-year-old male technician

History   For more than 10 years, xanthelasmata palpebralia, which were treated with trichloro-acetic acid; for 5 years, tumors of the finger tendons and hypercholesterolemia have been present.

Physical Examination   On the extensor tendons of digits II, III, and IV, yellow subcutaneous tumors, varying from round to longitudinal, 1.2 cm in diameter. Moreover, similar tumors in the Achilles tendon and the tendons under the feet; on the right superior eyelid and both inferior eyelids there are yellow streaks.

Differential Diagnosis   Tendinous and palpebral xanthomata in hyperlipoproteinemia, probably type II[a] or II[b]

Blood Chemistry   Serum clear. Total lipids: 1316 mg per 100 ml.[1] Total cholesterols: 523 mg per 100 ml.[1] Triglycerides: 115 mg per 100 ml. Low-density (beta) lipoproteins: 1053 mg per 100 ml.[2] Very low density (pre-beta) lipoproteins: 132 mg per 100 ml.

Clues   Clinical picture and blood chemistry

Treatment and Course   Treatment with low-caloric, low-fat, and low-cholesterol diet, at times combined with cholestyramine and nicotinic acid derivatives, did not significantly influence the lipid content of the serum nor the xanthomata. During the 10-year observation period, the patient developed a myocardial infarction.

Significance   Clear serum, elevated cholesterol due to elevated LDL, elevated total lipids, and normal triglycerides are characteristic for type II[a] familial hyperlipoproteinemia, which is often complicated by xanthomata of eyelids and tendons and cardiovascular disease. This type is very resistant to therapy.

---

[1] Elevated.
[2] Markedly elevated.

Xanthoma Tuberosum

This comprises yellowish-purple nodules located especially on the elbows and knees and occurs in patients with type II, III, IV, or V pattern.

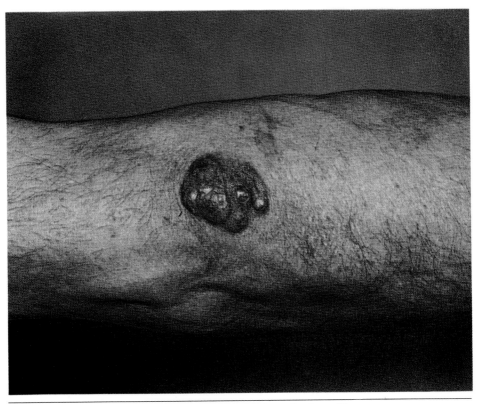

56 Xanthomata tuberosa in hyperlipoproteinemia, type III

Patient Profile *Forty-two-year-old truck driver*

History *For 7 years, excrescences on the left elbow and for 2 years on the right elbow also. Is overweight: height is 1.87 m; weight is 97.6 kg*

Physical Examination *On the left elbow, a conglomeration of yellow-violet tumors with a total diameter of 3 cm. Similar tumors on the right elbow. In the palms, yellow creases. No ASCVD.*

Differential Diagnosis *Tuberous xanthomata caused by hyperlipoproteinemia.*

Histopathology *In the dermis, groups of foam cells*

Laboratory Examinations *Urine: albumin and reduction negative. Serum: turbid. Total lipids: 1529 mg per 100 ml.[1] Total sterol: 422 mg per 100 ml.[1] Triglycerides: 503 mg per 100 ml. Low-density lipoproteins: 413 mg per 100 ml. Very low density lipoproteins: 963 mg per 100 ml.[1] Cholesterol/triglycerides ratio in VLDL: 0.68.[1]*

Clues *Clinical aspect, elevated total cholesterol and triglyceride levels in blood, presence of β-VLDL.*

Treatment *Low-carbohydrate, low-caloric, sugar-free diet, resulting in lowering of the total lipids until total lipids were 917 mg per 100 ml, triglycerides 246 mg per 100 ml, total cholesterol 218 mg per 100 ml, and disappearance of the xanthomata*

---

[1] Elevated.

Xanthoma Eruptivum (Eruptive Xanthoma)

These discrete inflammatory-type papules "erupt" suddenly and in showers, appearing typically on the buttocks.

ETIOLOGY

Characteristically associated with diabetes mellitus but also with other disorders (see Table B) and with type III hyperlipoproteinemia

HISTORY

Lesions may be tender

PHYSICAL EXAMINATION

Skin Lesions

TYPE

Papules, discrete
Nodules represent confluent papules

COLOR   Yellow center with red halo
SHAPE   Dome-shaped

ARRANGEMENT

Scattered discrete lesions in a localized region (e.g., buttocks)
"Tight" clusters and may become confluent to form "tuberoeruptive" xanthomata

DISTRIBUTION

Papules: buttocks, elbows, knees, back, or anywhere
"Tuberoeruptive" lesions: elbows (often seen with xanthoma striatum palmaris associated with type III)

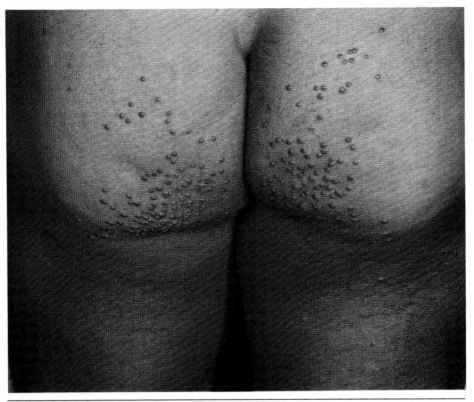

57　Xanthomata papuloeruptiva in type IV hyperlipoproteinemia and diabetes

Patient Profile　Forty-three-year-old taxi driver

History　For 2 years, intermittent claudication and diabetes. Patient did not adhere to his diet. A few months previously, yellow nodules developed on the buttocks, arms, and trunk. Patient was overweight and an alcoholic.

Physical Examination　Regionally disseminated discrete yellow papules, 1 to 3 mm in diameter, on the buttocks. Similar papules on the arms and trunk.

Histopathology　In the dermis, nests of foam cells. Oil red O staining: positive. Electron microscopy: "lipid inclusions" in the melanocytes

Blood Chemistry　Blood sugar: 15.8 mmol per 100 ml.[1] Serum: very turbid. Total lipids: 4286 mg per 100 ml.[2] Total cholesterol: 900 mg per 100 ml.[2] Triglycerides 2186 mg per 100 ml.[3] LDL: 300 mg per 100 ml. VLDL: 3386 mg per 100 ml.[2] Ratio cholesterol/triglycerides in VLDL: 0.37.

Clues　Clinical picture, elevated blood sugar, elevation of total cholesterol, relatively higher elevation of triglycerides.

Treatment and Prognosis　Low-carbohydrate, low-alcohol, low-caloric diet. After 4 months, disappearance of the xanthomata, total lipids = 1362 mg per 100 ml,[1] total cholesterols = 298 mg per 100 ml, triglycerides = 588 mg per 100 ml.[1]

[1] Elevated.
[2] Markedly elevated.
[3] Very markedly elevated.

Xanthoma Striatum Palmare

Xanthomata striata palmaria exhibit yellow-orange, flat or slightly elevated infiltrations of the creases of the palms and fingers. This is highly characteristic for type III hyperlipoproteinemia but is also seen in obstructive biliary disease and dysglobulinemia.

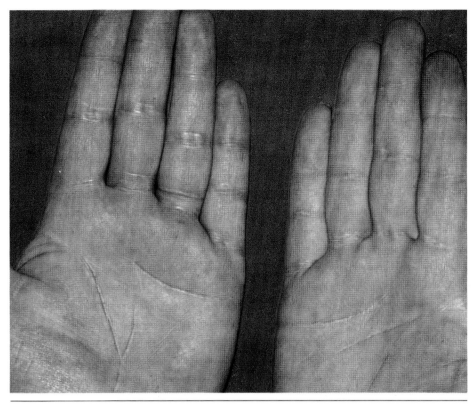

58 Xanthomata striata palmaria in type III hyperlipoproteinemia

Patient Profile *Fifty-one-year-old female homemaker*

History *For 5 months, yellow streaks in the palms and yellow excrescences on the elbows*

Physical Examination *The creases of the palms are yellow. The palmar creases of the meta-carpophalangeal and interphalangeal joints show elevated yellow streaks. There are discrete yellow papules on the elbows, buttocks, and knees. No ASCVD.*

Laboratory Examinations *Blood sugar: normal. Serum: moderately turbid. Total lipids: 2816 mg per 100 ml.[1] Total cholesterol: 743 mg per 100 ml.[2] Triglycerides: 863 mg per 100 ml.[2] LDL: 338 mg per 100 ml. VLDL: 2140 mg per 100 ml.[2] Ratio of cholesterol to triglycerides in VLDL: 0.8.[1]*

Clues *Clinical picture, triglycerides relatively more enhanced than total cholesterol, presence of β-VLDL.*

Treatment *Low-caloric, low-carbohydrate, sugar-free diet with 40 percent fat. The xanthoma disappeared in 1 year; patient's weight was reduced to 64.4 kg, the total lipids to 918, and the total cholesterol to 260.*

Significance *Hyperlipoproteinemia caused by elevated VLDL is classified as type III when the ratio of cholesterol to triglycerides in VLDL is greater than 0.5. Clinically distinctive are palmar linear xanthomata and xanthochromia striata. Early diagnosis and treatment may prevent ASCVD.*

---

[1] Elevated.
[2] Markedly elevated.

Vitiligo

Vitiligo is an idiopathic, acquired, usually patterned, circumscribed hypomelanosis of skin and hair in which other causes of hypomelanosis (postinflammation, chemical, etc.) have been excluded; there is an absence of melanocytes in fully developed hypomelanotic vitiligo macules. The disease is important not only because the disfigurement can result in psychologic problems, especially in brown and black patients, but because it may be a marker for thyroid disease and less frequently certain other diseases.

EPIDEMIOLOGY

Sex and Race Reported female predominance is probably related to selective concern with disfigurement rather than to true incidence. More obvious in persons with dark skin but probably not more prevalent. Family history in 30% of patients.

Incidence One percent (range, 0.14 to 8.8%)

Skin Phototypes Mostly Types III, IV, V, and VI (less apparent in Skin Phototypes I and II)

HISTORY

Age of Onset Infancy to old age; peak incidence is 10 to 30 years (congenital vitiligo is very rare)

Precipitating Factors Physical trauma

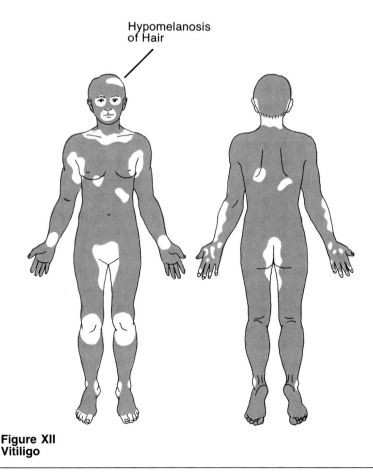

Hypomelanosis of Hair

Figure XII
Vitiligo

(Koebner or isomorphic phenomenon), severe sunburn, sites of surgical scars; following abrasions; pressure sites such as the belt-line and bra straps; following emotional stress

PHYSICAL EXAMINATION

Skin Lesions

TYPE Macule, sharply marginated, no epidermal change (i.e., scale or atrophy)
COLOR Typically pure "snow white," but newly developing areas "off-white" or tan; margins often hyperpigmented
SHAPE Oval, geographic patterns
DISTRIBUTION
Focal Isolated macule or macules in one site
Segmental Unilateral, quasidermatomal
Generalized (see Figure XII) Multiple discrete macules, often symmetrical (even mirror image) and at sites of repeated trauma (elbows, knees, ankles)
Universal Total loss of melanin in all the skin, in most of the hair, but not the eyes
Hair Pigmented or depigmented hairs may be present in a vitiligo macule; white streaks in scalp, eyelashes, beard hair
Eye Examination Iritis in 10% or more, may not be clearly symptomatic; changes consistent with healed chorioretinitis in up to 30%

LABORATORY AND SPECIAL EXAMINATIONS

Dermatopathology and Electron Microscopy

SITE Epidermis. No changes except absence of melanocytes; at the margin of the white macules there may be large melanocytes, and a few lymphocytes. In an atypical presentation of white macules a biopsy for light microscopy is necessary. In vitiligo, chemical leukoderma, and piebaldism, melanocytes are absent but in the white macules of tuberous sclerosis and nevus depigmentosus, melanocytes are present.
BLOOD CHEMISTRY Rule out thyroid disease (T_4, TSH); over 40% of patients, particularly women, with vitiligo over 50 years of age have thyroid disease: hypo- or hyperthyroidism. CBC with indices (PA), Na, K (Addison's disease) for individuals with strong family history of vitiligo and vitiligo-associated diseases

WOOD'S LAMP This is necessary to detect the lesions in fair-skinned patients.
EYE EXAMINATION Necessary in all patients (see "Eye" findings) by an ophthalmologist

DIFFERENTIAL DIAGNOSIS

Lupus erythematosus must be excluded in atypical presentations (history, physical examination, biopsy, immunofluorescence, and ANA). Other causes of circumscribed hypomelanosis include: *pityriasis alba* (not sharp margins, slight scaling), *tinea versicolor* (potassium hydroxide examination), *piebaldism* (lesions present at birth, large dark hyperpigmented macules within the white areas, white forelock), *chemical leukoderma* (history of exposure to phenolic germicides), *leprosy* (white areas are anesthetic), *nevus depigmentosus* (stable, not amelanotic, unlike segmental vitiligo, melanocytes present on biopsy).

PATHOPHYSIOLOGY

An immune hypothesis appears feasible. This would involve an aberration of immune surveillance that results in destruction of melanocytes; the primary event would be injury to melanocytes with release of antigen and subsequent autoimmunization (probably in a genetically predisposed individual).

PROGNOSIS

Without treatment, the white macules remain stable or enlarge; new white areas may appear until the total skin is white. With oral PUVA photochemotherapy or therapeutic depigmentation, the results are good to excellent. (See Treatment)
About 30% have some degree of spontaneous repigmentation but usually in a few macules only, and rarely cosmetically satisfactory.

TREATMENT

Sunscreens SPF 15 clear or creamy preparations. Particularly important for sun-exposed areas of the face, arms, and hands to prevent acute and chronic effects of UV radiation, including koebnerization
Cosmetic Coverup Makeups: Dermablend (Flori Roberts), Covermark

(Lydia O'Leary). Dyes: Dy O-Derm (Owen Labs), Vita Dye (Elder).

Repigmentation

Topical corticosteroids (e.g., clobetasol-17-propionate) used for only 6 to 8 weeks are occasionally effective for small macules and are helpful, especially in children. Since telangiectasia, atrophy, and strias may develop, regular monitoring by a dermatologist is required.

Topical 8-methoxypsoralen (8-MOP) may be used in carefully selected patients; application of the 0.1% 8-MOP solution or ointment (petrolatum) followed by controlled UVA exposures indoors once weekly. Topical psoralens are extremely phototoxic, and this treatment should be done by a physician with experience using this method.

Oral photochemotherapy may be helpful in up to 70% of carefully selected vitiligo patients. Schedules include 0.3–0.6 mg/kg 8-MOP plus artificial UVA, or 0.6–0.9 mg/kg trimethylpsoralen (TMP) plus sunlight or artificial UVA systems. Treat only patients over age 12 (when eyes are adequately mature) and insist on eye protection outdoors at least 24 hours after therapy. Treatments are given twice weekly, not 2 days in a row. Response begins in 15 to 25 treatments and requires 100 to 300 or more to satisfactory conclusion. Face and neck have a 60 to 70% response rate; trunk, arms, and legs nearly as good, but dorsal areas of the hands and feet respond poorly. Fully repigmented macules have an 85% retention rate. Good patient compliance and careful physician supervision seem part of the formula for success.

Depigmentation Benoquin (20% monobenzylether of hydroquinone) is indicated in patients who have tried or failed with PUVA and who can accept the irreversible nature of this method of treatment. Relative criteria include (1) age over 40, and (2) over 40% involvement of the body with vitiligo. Application is twice daily. Transient irritation is common but contact dermatitis is uncommon. Treatment requires a year or more to complete. Depigmentation may not be confined to sites of application but can appear in remote areas. Leukotrichia is a rare complication. Depigmentation is expected to be permanent and irreversible. Occasional reappearance of pigmented macules may sometimes occur on exposed areas, but reapplication of Benoquin for a month or two will cause a regression. Patients who have been completely depigmented can achieve a more normal appearance with oral beta carotene.

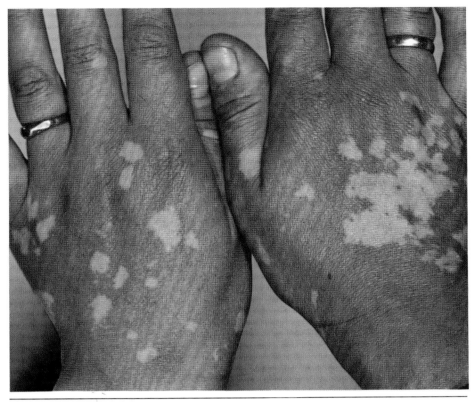

59 Vitiligo

Patient Profile Thirty-two-year-old female homemaker

History For a year, gradually enlarging white spots

Physical Examination On the dorsa of the hands, irregularly disseminated, in part confluent, hypopigmented macules; similar lesions on the feet and trunk

Differential Diagnosis Pityriasis versicolor

Laboratory and Special Examinations Examination for Malassezia furfur (Pityrosporum ovale) negative

Neurofibromatosis

This important autosomal dominant neurocutaneous disorder is manifested by changes in cells derived from the neural crest: *skin melanocytes* (café-au-lait macules), *eye melanocytes* (Lish nodules in the iris), *Schwann cells* (neurofibroma), *adrenal medulla* (pheochromocytoma), and *leptomeninges* (meningioma). Two forms of neurofibromatosis appear to exist: (1) classical *Von Recklinghausen's neurofibromatosis* now called neurofibromatosis-1 (NF-1); as first described in 1882 and which affects 80,000 persons in the United States; and (2) *central or acoustic neurofibromatosis* now called neurofibromatosis-2 (NF-2). Both types may have café-au-lait macules and neurofibromas, but only the central type has *bilateral* acoustic neuromas (*unilateral* acoustic neuromas are a variable feature of VRN). Another feature present in VRN but not present in the central or acoustic type are Lisch nodules (pigmented hamartomas in the iris), which occur in 92 percent of patients with VRN *over the age of 16 years.*

EPIDEMIOLOGY AND ETIOLOGY

Age

Café-au-lait macules appear in infancy, rarely congenital
Neurofibromata appear during late childhood in increasing numbers
Acoustic neuromas in teenagers and young adults

Sex Males more than females
Heredity Autosomal dominant, NF-1 on chromosome 17
Incidence NF-1, 1:4,000; NF-2, 1:50,000

HISTORY

Duration of Lesions See above
Skin Symptoms None, except tenderness and pain in some neurofibromata
Systems Review Symptoms reflecting various organ involvement: deafness (acoustic neuroma), hypertensive headaches (pheochromocytoma), pathologic fractures (bone cysts), mental retardation (60 percent), brain tumor (astrocytoma)

PHYSICAL EXAMINATION

Skin Lesions See Figure 60.
TYPE

Café-au-lait macules Present in normal population 10 to 20 percent, 0.5 to 1.5 cm, fewer than three. Critical number for suspicion of neurofibromatosis:

Under 5 years: five or more greater than 0.5 cm
Over 5 years: six or more greater than 1.5 cm

"Freckles" In axillae are highly correlated but not pathognomonic
Nodules Skin-colored or brown, pedunculated, soft or firm (see Figure 60)
Plexiform neuromas Drooping, soft, doughy
DISTRIBUTION Random and generalized or rarely localized to one region
Other Physical Findings Lisch nodules (pigmented) in the iris,[1] increased blood pressure, kyphosis, elephantiasis neuromatosa (gross disfigurement from neurofibromatosis of the nerve trunks)

DIAGNOSIS

Tentative Criteria for the Diagnosis of von Recklinghausen's Neurofibromatosis[2]

1. Café-au-lait macules >6 lesions with diameter of 1.5 cm or more (adults) *or* >5 lesions with diameter of 0.5 or more (younger than 5 years of age) and melanin macroglobules, >10 per 5 high-power fields in "split" dopa specimens (white adults)
2. Axillary or inguinal freckling
3. Pigmented nodules of the iris (Lisch nodules) > 2
4. Cutaneous neurofibromata (>2) or one plexiform neurofibroma
5. A first-degree relative (parent, sibling, or child) with NF-1

---

[1]The prevalence of Lisch nodules increases with age. Lisch nodules are not found in normal persons and are visualized by binocular biomicroscopy and proximal rather than direct illumination. They are seen as "glassy" translucent papules up to 2.0 mm—tan and dome-shaped.
[2]Any one of the two.

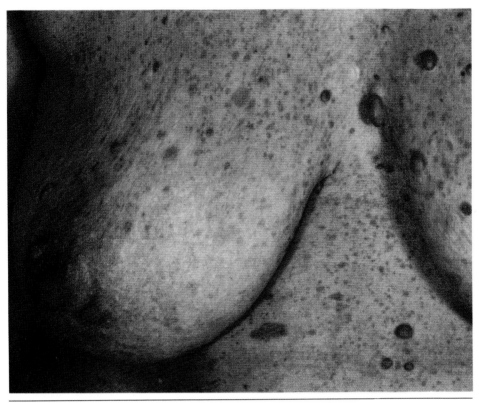

60 Neurofibromatosis (Von Recklinghausen's disease)

Patient Profile *Forty-six-year-old female*

History *For 30 years, numerous soft tumors and a large number of brown spots disseminated over the body. No other physical or mental complaints. Family history: noncontributory.*

Physical Examination *On the trunk and extremities, many soft, flesh-colored or violaceous papules and nodules, varying in size from a few millimeters to a centimeter. Some are pedunculated, others lobulate. On pressure, "button holing" phenomenon. In addition, several café-au-lait spots. Neurologic examination: no abnormalities.*

Differential Diagnosis *Multiple pedunculated fibromas*

Laboratory and Special Examinations *Biopsy from tumor: in dermis, dense wavy fibrils of young collagen and occasionally mucoid degeneration. Café au-lait spots: (EM) melanin macroglobules in basal cells of epidermis.*

6. Optic glioma
7. Sphenoid dysplasia or thinning of long bone cortex with or without pseudoarthrosis

COURSE AND PROGNOSIS

Variable involvement over time from only café-au-lait macules to marked disfigurement with thousands of nodules. Close follow-up for malignancy in NF-1 patients.

Ichthyosis Vulgaris (Dominant and X-linked)

Ichthyosis vulgaris is a genetic disorder of keratinization leading to dry, scaly skin.

GENERAL REMARKS

Two clinically and histologically distinct types of ichthyosis vulgaris are now recognized: dominant ichthyosis vulgaris (DIV) (with an incidence of 1:300) and a rarer form (1:6000), sex-linked ichthyosis vulgaris.

Dominant Ichthyosis Vulgaris

EPIDEMIOLOGY AND ETIOLOGY

Age Not congenital, develops in 1 to 4 years
Sex No differences
General May be associated with atopy

HISTORY

Skin Symptoms Winter pruritus, irritation, and roughness of skin

PHYSICAL EXAMINATION

Skin Lesions

TYPE

Xeroderma (dry skin) with fine white scaling
Follicular keratosis (so-called keratosis pilaris)
Increased creases of palms and soles

COLOR Normal skin color (compare X-linked ichthyosis)
SHAPE Fish-scale pattern, especially on the shins (see Figure 61)
DISTRIBUTION (see Figure XIII)

Diffuse involvement, accentuated on the shins, arms, and back, but sparing the axillae and the fossae (antecubital and popliteal)
Follicular keratosis: arms, buttocks, thighs

Eye Lesions Keratopathy (rare)

DERMATOPATHOLOGY

Site—epidermis. There is hyperkeratosis but a reduced or absent granular layer; the germinative layer is flattened.

COURSE

May show improvement in the summer and in adulthood

TREATMENT

Hydration by immersion in bath and oils plus emollients.
Newer agents that bind water or control scaling include alpha-hydroxy acid-lactic acid. Also creams and ointments containing urea (10–25%) accomplish the same result.

X-linked Ichthyosis Vulgaris

EPIDEMIOLOGY

Age Appearance at birth or in infancy

CLINICAL FEATURES

Different than DIV Large brown scales; involves the sides of neck, antecubital and popliteal fossae, and the chest and abdomen; *normal* palms and soles; scalp scaling is sometimes prominent; no follicular keratoses
Eye Involvement Stromal corneal opacities more frequent than in DIV, developing in the second or third decade

COURSE

No improvement with age

TREATMENT

Same as for dominant ichthyosis vulgaris

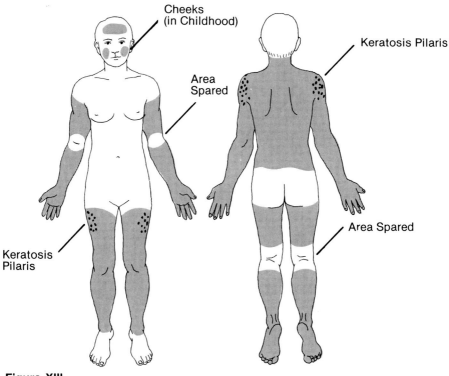

Figure XIII
Ichthyosis Vulgaris (Dominant)

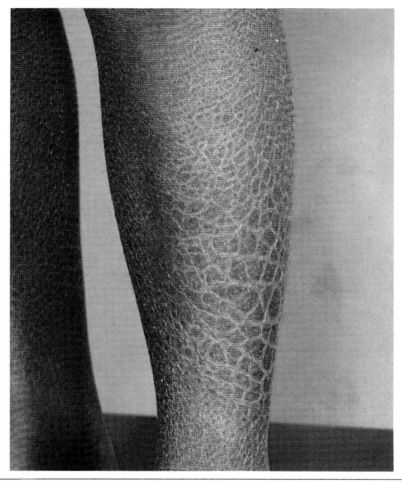

61 Ichthyosis vulgaris

Patient Profile Twenty-five-year-old student

History Since youth, gradually more pronounced "dry" skin. Several relatives have the same complaint.

Physical Examination Hyperkeratotic scaling predominantly on the flanks, arms, and lower legs. The skin of the elbows, axillae, and knee folds is smooth.

Differential Diagnosis Other types of ichthyosis

Treatment Maintenance treatment with 10% urea-containing creams

Impetigo

This is an acute purulent infection which is at first vesicular and later crusted—a very superficial infection of the skin due to group A streptococci and often *Staphylococcus aureus,* or a mixed infection.

EPIDEMIOLOGY AND ETIOLOGY

Age Preschool children and young adults
Predisposing Factors Crowded living conditions, poor hygiene, and neglected minor trauma. "Impetiginization" also occurs on lesions of eczema and scabies. It is important to obtain cultures of household and other close contacts, and those that are positive should be treated.

HISTORY

Duration of Lesions Days
Skin Symptoms Variable pruritus

PHYSICAL EXAMINATION

Skin Lesions

TYPE

Transient thin-roofed vesicles →
crusts
Erosions

COLOR Golden-yellow "stuck on" crusts (see Figure 62)
SIZE AND SHAPE 1.0 to 3.0 cm; round or oval; central healing
ARRANGEMENT Scattered discrete lesions, some large confluent lesions; satellite lesions occur by autoinoculation
DISTRIBUTION Face, arms, legs
Miscellaneous Physical Findings Regional lymphadenopathy

DIFFERENTIAL DIAGNOSIS

In the early vesicular stage impetigo may simulate *varicella* and *herpes simplex.* *Tinea corporis* with central clearing and pustules shows mycelia.

LABORATORY AND SPECIAL EXAMINATIONS

Gram Stain of Early Vesicle Gram-positive cocci, in chains or clusters, may be present.
Culture Group A streptococci and sometimes a mixed culture of streptococci and *S. aureus* (especially from older lesions). Use of a moistened culture swab to dissolve crusts may be necessary to isolate the pathogens.

TREATMENT (see Appendix G)

1. Penicillin, single injection of long-acting benzathine penicillin. Penicillin V in divided doses for 10 days.
2. If staphylococci are present, dicloxacillin or cloxacillin (2 g per day in four divided doses for 10 days).
3. Erythromycin administered for 10 days. This is used if patient cannot take penicillins.

COMPLICATIONS

Glomerulonephritis with certain streptococcal strains

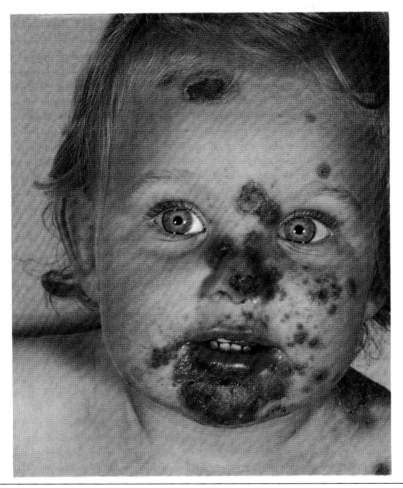

62 Impetigo vulgaris

Patient Profile Two-year-old female

History Nonpruritic eruption on the face and trunk, present for 1 week

Physical Examination On the face and shoulder, scattered, discrete, sharply demarcated crusts and erosions, mostly round, some confluent

Differential Diagnosis Infected eczema

Microbiologic Examination Bacterial culture from eroded surface: Group A streptococcus—sensitive to all antibiotics. S. aureus hemolyticus—sensitive to all antibiotics.

Clues Crusts, absence of pruritus and other symptoms of eczema, bacteriology

Bullous Impetigo (Staphylococcal Impetigo)

This form of impetigo occurs as scattered thin-walled bullae arising in normal skin and containing clear yellow or slightly turbid fluid without surrounding erythema.

EPIDEMIOLOGY AND ETIOLOGY

Age Neonates or older children
Predisposing Factors This may occur in epidemic form in infant nurseries
Etiology Phage II staphylococci, which produce an extracellular exotoxin, and which also produce, besides bullous impetigo, exfoliative disease (staphylococcal scalded-skin syndrome)

PHYSICAL EXAMINATION

Skin Lesions

TYPE Vesicles and bullae (see Figure 63): thin-walled, easily ruptured, without surrounding erythema, and which contain clear light to dark yellow fluid
ARRANGEMENT Scattered discrete lesions
DISTRIBUTION Trunk

DIFFERENTIAL DIAGNOSIS

Bullous varicella (which probably represents superinfection of varicella with phage II staphylococci)

LABORATORY EXAMINATION

Gram stain of early vesicle: gram-positive cocci

TREATMENT (see Appendix I)

Nafcillin, 50 to 100 mg/kg per day in divided doses every 4 to 6 hr, and at a dose of 100 to 200 mg/kg every 4 to 6 hr for older children
Sheets and towels should be changed daily
Bacitracin or mupirocin should be used in the nostrils and applied to the lesions

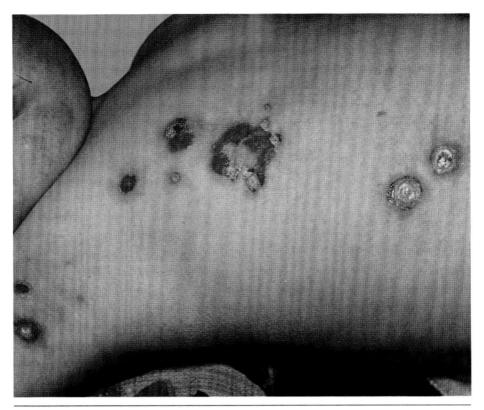

63 Impetigo contagiosa

Patient Profile Fifteen-month-old male

History For 5 days, an eruption on the trunk and axillary fold; no pruritus

Physical Examination Disseminated over trunk and axilla are round and serpiginous, sharply demarcated lesions. Several are only red and erosive; others are covered by a thin, white to yellow crust.

Laboratory and Special Examinations Staphylococcus aureus hemolyticus, coagulase-positive and insensitive to penicillin; sensitive for streptomycin, chloramphenicol, erythromycin, and tetracycline. Streptococcus viridans sensitive to all tested antibiotics.

Clues Sharply demarcated lesions, absence of pruritus, bacterial culture

Ulcerative Impetigo (Ecthyma)

This is a confusing term that usually refers to an ulcerative bacterial infection caused most frequently by group A streptococci or staphylococci, or both.

EPIDEMIOLOGY AND ETIOLOGY

Age Children, adolescents, elderly

Predisposing Factors Lesion of neglect—develops in excoriations; insect bites; minor trauma in elderly patients, soldiers, and alcoholics

HISTORY

Duration of Lesions Weeks

Skin Symptoms Pruritic and tender

PHYSICAL EXAMINATION

Skin Lesions

TYPE Vesicle or pustule → ulcer: raised border, violaceous

COLOR Dirty yellowish gray crust (see Figure 64)

SHAPE AND SIZE Round or oval, 0.5 to 3.0 cm

PALPATION Indurated

ARRANGEMENT Scattered, discrete

SITES OF PREDILECTION Ankles, dorsa of feet, thighs, buttocks

LABORATORY AND SPECIAL EXAMINATIONS

Culture Group A streptococci, staphylococci

TREATMENT

Several weeks of antibiotic treatment with penicillin or erythromycin. Lesions heal with a scar.

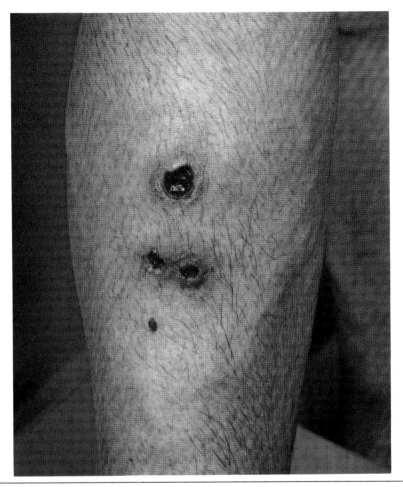

64 Ecthyma

Patient Profile *Seventeen-year-old boy*

History *For 6 weeks, on the lower legs three lesions that started as red-crusted patches with ulcerations*

Physical Examination *Over the tibia are three well-demarcated ulcers, in part surrounded by a small erythematous area. The bottom of the ulcers is not necrotic.*

Differential Diagnosis *Slowly healing wounds, leishmaniasis, reaction to insect bites, pyoderma*

Laboratory and Special Examinations *Gram stain of exudate: abundant cocci and polymorpho-nuclear leukocytes. Culture for bacteria:* Streptococcus pyogenes, *group A. This was also found in the nose.*

Clues *"Punched out" ulcers on legs and arms of short duration whether or not covered by crusts, demonstration of pathogenic cocci (*Streptococcus pyogenes, *group A, or , less common,* Staphylococcus aureus)

Superficial Folliculitis

This superficial inflammation of hair follicles, often bacterial, heals without scarring.

EPIDEMIOLOGY AND ETIOLOGY

Occupation Contact with mineral oils
Predisposing Factors Exposure to tar, adhesive plaster, plastic occlusive dressings. *Staphylococcus aureus* folliculitis aggravated by shaving, i.e., beard area, axillae, legs

HISTORY

Duration of Lesions Days
Skin Symptoms Usually nontender or slightly tender; may be pruritic
Constitutional Symptoms None

PHYSICAL EXAMINATION

Skin Lesions

TYPE Pustule confined to the ostium of the hair follicle
COLOR Dirty yellow or gray with erythema
ARRANGEMENT Scattered discrete or more frequently grouped
DISTRIBUTION

Face Folliculitis (sycosis) barbae due to staphylococcal infection (see Figure 65)
Scalp or legs Follicular impetigo of Bockhart (see Figure 66)
Trunk Pseudomonas aeruginosa ("hot tub") folliculitis

Back Candida albicans in febrile hospitalized patients; pustular miliaria, etc.

LABORATORY FINDINGS

Gram stain: look for gram-positive cocci in clusters within PMN
Staphylococcus aureus, Candida albicans, Pseudomonas aeruginosa

DIFFERENTIAL DIAGNOSIS

Beard area: acne, flat warts, molluscum contagiosum, tinea barbi
Tinea corporis (presence of mycelia in direct preparation); *pustular miliaria,* not perifollicular (occurs in hot and humid weather)

TREATMENT

Remove exciting agent (e.g., tar, mineral oils)
Topical antibacterial agents
Systemic antibiotic for sycosis barbae (see Appendix I)
Oxacillin or dicloxacillin
If allergic to penicillin: erythromycin should be used
If *Staphylococcus aureus* is cultured from the nostrils, daily application of mupirocin should be started

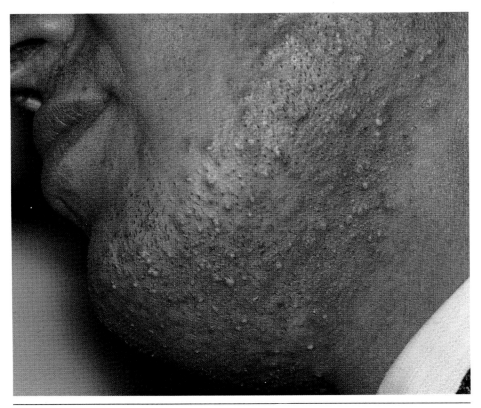

65 Sycosis barbae (bacterial)

Patient Profile   Thirty-year-old male office worker

History   For 2 years, a recurrent eruption in the beard region

Physical Examination   Numerous pustules and few papules in the whole beard region in a follicular arrangement

Laboratory and Special Examinations   Staphylococcus aureus hemolyticus, coagulase-positive, sensitive to all tested antibiotics

Clues   Bacterial culture, clinical aspect, absence of ingrown hairs

Prognosis and Significance   Since the introduction of corticosteroids and antibiotics, the prognosis is good.

---

[1] N.B.: Not used in the United States.

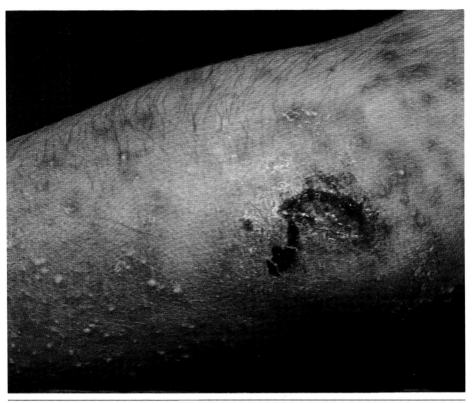

66 Superficial folliculitis

Patient Profile Eight-year-old boy

History A few days previous, trauma of the left elbow resulted in a deep excoriation. Under a wet dressing applied by the patient, a rapidly spreading pustular eruption appeared.

Physical Examination An oval excoriation, 3 by 1.5 cm, with a red floor and blood crusts. In the surrounding area, disseminated in a follicular pattern, pinpoint to large pustules, some with a vellus hair in the middle. No pruritus.

Differential Diagnosis Acute eczema

Laboratory and Special Examinations Excoriation and floor of the ulcer: Staphylococcus aureus hemolyticus, coagulase-positive. Sensitive to penicillin and all other tested antibiotics.

Clues Clinical aspect and bacterial culture

Pathophysiology Under the moist environment of the wet dressing the bacteria on the skin proliferated and infected the uppermost part of the hair follicle.

Furuncle

A furuncle is an acute, deep-seated, red, hot, very tender, inflammatory nodule that evolves from a staphylococcal folliculitis.

EPIDEMIOLOGY AND ETIOLOGY

Age Children, adolescents, and young adults
Sex More common in boys
Predisposing Factors Chronic staphylococcal carrier state in nares or perineum, friction of collars or belts, obesity, bactericidal defects (e.g., in chronic granulomatosis), defects in chemotaxis and hyper-IgE, diabetes mellitus. May complicate scabies, pediculosis, or abrasions.

HISTORY

Duration of Lesions Days
Skin Symptoms Throbbing pain and invariable exquisite tenderness
Constitutional Symptoms Not infrequently low-grade fever and malaise

PHYSICAL EXAMINATION

Skin Lesions

TYPE Hard nodule, then fluctuant, then ruptures into an ulcer, with erythematous halo (see Figures 67 and 68)
COLOR Bright red
PALPATION Indurated
SHAPE Round
ARRANGEMENT Scattered, discrete
DISTRIBUTION Isolated single lesions or a few multiple lesions
SITES OF PREDILECTION Occur only where there are hair follicles and in areas subject to friction and sweating: nose, neck, face, axillae, buttocks, or paronychia

SPECIAL STUDIES

Culture of blood in cases with fever and/or constitutional symptoms before beginning treatment; if blood culture is positive, intravenous antibiotics are necessary.
Aspiration of pustules for Gram stain, culture and antibiotic sensitivity studies.

DIFFERENTIAL DIAGNOSIS

Necrotic herpes simplex, hidradenitis suppurativa (in axillae, groin, vulva; presence of double comedones)

TREATMENT (see Appendix I for doses of antibiotics)

Simple furunculosis is treated by local application of heat. No systemic antibiotics are needed except in patients at risk for bacteremia (e.g., immunosuppressed patients).
Furunculosis with surrounding cellulitis or with fever should be treated with systemic antibiotics such as cloxacillin or with erythromycin. Treatment should continue for 1 week; incision and drainage is commonly required.
Recurrent furunculosis may be difficult to control. This may be related to persistent staphylococci in the nares, perineum, and body folds. Effective control can sometimes be obtained with frequent showers (not baths) with providone-iodine soap and antibacterial ointments (mupirocin) applied daily to the inside of the nares.

COMPLICATIONS

May occur with severe furunculosis and carbuncle formation. Bacteremia with hematogenous dissemination to heart valves, joints, spine, long bones, and viscera (especially kidneys)

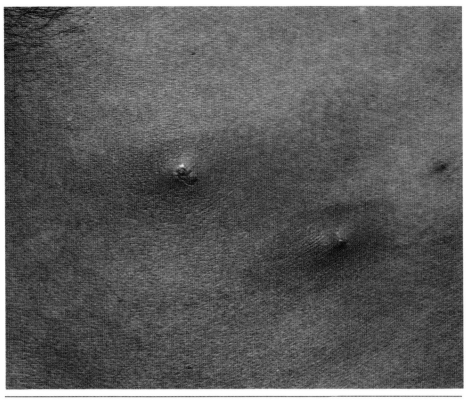

67 Furuncle

Patient Profile   Forty-five-year-old garage mechanic

History   For a week, pustules disseminated on trunk and upper arm. Patient was afebrile.

Physical Examination   Papules, 3 mm in diameter with central necrosis and a red margin of approximately 1 cm, disseminated, without a characteristic pattern

Laboratory and Special Examinations   Bacterial culture from the pustule and from the vestibulum nasi: Staphylococcus aureus hemolyticus, coagulase-positive. Sensitive for all tested antibiotics.

Treatment   Hot wet packs, topical antibiotics. Treatment of the nose with antibiotic cream. Cleared in a month.

Significance   Persons working with mineral oil are prone to skin infections.

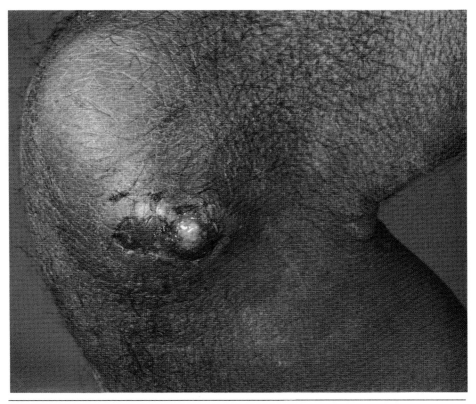

68   Furuncle

Patient Profile   *Fifty-eight-year-old farmer*

History   *For a few days, on both arms and left hand, painful infiltrations discharging pus*

Physical Examination   *On the right elbow, a red, painful, elevated, fluctuating infiltration 4 cm in diameter; in the center, a crater 0.8 cm in diameter containing a yellow mass. Similar lesions on left hand and axilla. No temperature elevation.*

Laboratory and Special Examinations   *Bacteriologic ulcer:* Staphylococcus aureus *hemolyticus, coagulase-positive. Nose: same bacteria as furuncle. Both insensitive to penicillin; sensitive to other antibiotics*

Erysipelas

Erysipelas is an acute infection of the dermis and hypodermis caused by *Streptococcus pyogenes,* group A, and characterized by rapid radial advancement via the lymphatics.

EPIDEMIOLOGY

Age Infants, young children, and older adults

HISTORY

Duration of Lesions Days (2 to 5) with abrupt onset

Skin Symptoms Pain and tenderness

Constitutional Symptoms

"ACUTE ILLNESS" SYNDROME Headaches, chills, fever, weakness
PREDISPOSING FACTORS Nephrotic edema, alcoholism, malnutrition, dysgammaglobulinemia, stasis dermatitis and lymphedema of the arm (postmastectomy with axillary node dissection) or of the calf (following coronary artery bypass using superficial veins of the leg)

PHYSICAL EXAMINATION

Appearance of Patient "Toxic"
Changes in Body Temperature Fever

Skin Lesions

TYPE Plaque, enlarging peripherally with advancing elevated sharp margin
COLOR Bright red (see Figure 69)
PALPATION Indurated lesion with "peau d'orange" appearance; warm to the touch
ARRANGEMENT Diffuse involvement of large area of skin surface (10 to 15 cm)
DISTRIBUTION Localized to one region (e.g., face)
SITES OF PREDILECTION Abdomen (infants); face, scalp, leg (older children); lower leg (half of adult patients); face (third of adult patients)

DIFFERENTIAL DIAGNOSIS

Herpes zoster (presence of pain prior to onset); *contact dermatitis* and *angioneurotic edema* (no fever or tenderness in the lesions); *Hemophilus influenzae* infection in young child

LABORATORY AND SPECIAL EXAMINATIONS

Culture Blood, throat, nose, eye may be positive for streptococcus; obtain culture with moistened cotton applicator at entry site
Serologic Test Increase in anti-DNAase 1 week after infection
Blood Studies Increase in polymorphonuclear cells (WBC: 15,000 to 40,000)

PATHOPHYSIOLOGY

Streptococci enter through a small break in the skin, such as a fissure or small puncture wound. The source of the infection is the upper respiratory tract. Postsurgical erysipelas is caused by transmittal of streptococci from nose, throat, or hands of the patient, nurse, or visitors.

TREATMENT (see Appendix I)

Penicillin V or, if patient is penicillin-sensitive or if organism is penicillin-resistant, erythromycin for 2 weeks. In acute erysipelas with negative blood cultures, intramuscular penicillin G, 1.2 million units every 6 hr; can be replaced by acid-resistant oral penicillin after 48 hr. Recurrences may occur in the same area.

COMPLICATIONS

Scarlet fever, streptococcal gangrene, fat necrosis, or coagulopathy

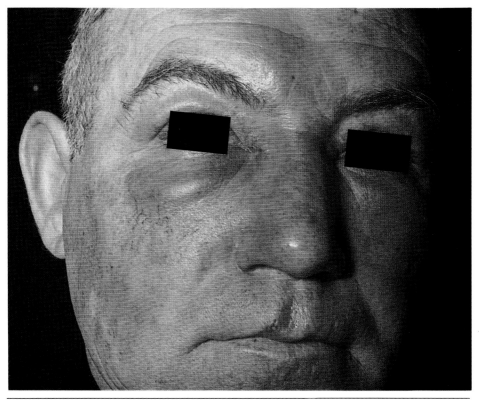

69 Erysipelas

Patient Profile Fifty-six-year-old male shopkeeper
History For 2 days, red swelling in the face. Temperature: 39.5°C.
Physical Examination Chiefly on the left cheek and extending over the nose and forehead, an erythematous swelling with a slightly elevated border, and edema of the eyelids
Laboratory and Special Examinations Leukocytosis: 15,500.
Clues Clinical aspect and fever

Erysipeloid

This acute infection of the hands is an occupational disease of people who fish and of butchers, caused by *Erysipelothrix insidiosa*.

ETIOLOGY

Occupation   Persons handling raw fish, fresh poultry, and meat products (butchers, fishers, cooks, veterinary surgeons)

HISTORY

Duration of Lesions   Days (2 to 7)
Skin Symptoms   Burning pain at site of injury, tender lesions
Constitutional Symptoms   Fever and malaise

PHYSICAL EXAMINATION

Skin Lesions

TYPE

Plaques with sharp margins which gradually enlarge centrifugally over a range of 10.0 cm, with central clearing
Vesicles, rarely, at the borders

COLOR   Characteristic violaceous (see Figure 70)
PALPATION   Warm, not hot, to touch
SHAPE   Irregular

ARRANGEMENT   Arciform border with central clearing
DISTRIBUTION   Localized
SITES OF PREDILECTION   Finger, hand, or forearm
Miscellaneous   Physical   Findings   Rarely, arthritis associated with the local lesion

DIFFERENTIAL DIAGNOSIS

The characteristic dusky red lesion on the hand or fingers is not like an acute cellulitis because it is not hot or very tender; also the history almost always pinpoints the incident and the source of infection.

LABORATORY AND SPECIAL EXAMINATIONS

Blood culture, as endocarditis may occur.
A culture of a biopsy may be helpful in identifying the organism.

TREATMENT

Penicillin in doses of *2 to 3 million units daily for 7 to 10 days* or erythromycin for an individual allergic to penicillin

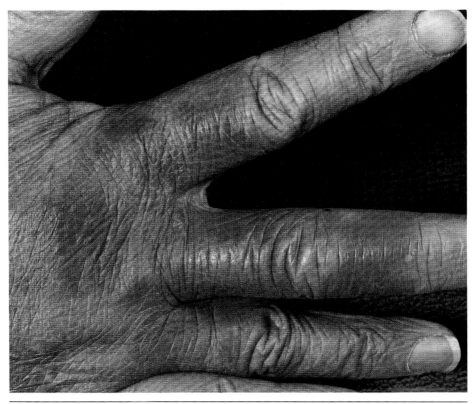

70 Erysipeloid

Patient Profile Forty-one-year-old fish handler

History For 8 days, a painful eruption of the fingers and back of the right hand. No elevation of temperature.

Physical Examination Red violaceous, sharply demarcated, slightly infiltrated macules 1 to 3 cm in diameter, irregularly disseminated over the backs of the fingers of the right hand

Differential Diagnosis Erysipelas

Clues Clinical picture, occupation, bacterial culture rarely possible

Pathophysiology Small wounds of the hands in butchers or fish handlers dealing with material contaminated by Erysipelothrix insidiosa

Treatment Cured after a course of penicillin

Erythrasma

Erythrasma (Greek, "red spot") is a chronic bacterial infection caused by *Corynebacterium minutissimum* affecting the intertriginous areas of the toes, groin, and axillae.

EPIDEMIOLOGY AND ETIOLOGY

Age Adults
Race Higher incidence in obese middle-aged blacks
Predisposing Factors Diabetes; warm, humid climate

HISTORY

Duration of Lesions Months, years
Skin Symptoms Irritation

PHYSICAL EXAMINATION

Skin Lesions

TYPE Scaling (fine) macules, sharply marginated (see Figure 71)
COLOR Red or brownish red (see Figure 71)
SHAPE Irregular, polycyclic
ARRANGEMENT Scattered discrete lesions, confluent patches
SITES OF PREDILECTION Groin, axillae, intergluteal, submammary

DIFFERENTIAL DIAGNOSIS

Tinea cruris (positive skin scrapings for hyphae), *seborrheic dermatitis* (negative preparations for organisms and absence of fluorescence)

LABORATORY AND SPECIAL EXAMINATIONS

Direct Microscopic Examination of Scales with Potassium Hydroxide (5%) Rods and filaments
Wood's Lamp Characteristic coral-red fluorescence

TREATMENT

Good clearing occurs with erythromycin, 250 mg qid for 14 days. Relapses usually occur within 6 months to a year. Topical antibacterial agents are not as effective. Miconazole or an imidazole cream is useful.

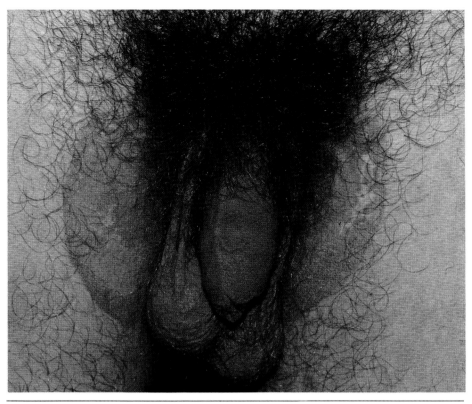

71 Erythrasma

Patient Profile Twenty-eight-year-old male

History For 3 months, slightly pruritic lesions on inner sides of thighs

Physical Examination On the inner sides of the thighs, adjacent to the scrotum, very sharply demarcated, diffuse, erythematous, light-brownish areas. On scratching, diffuse delicate scaling.

Differential Diagnosis Tinea, intertriginous eczema (intertrigo)

Laboratory and Special Examinations Direct microscopic examination of scrapings in 10% potassium hydroxide: rods and filaments. Gram-stained imprints of the horny layer: gram-positive rods. Wood's light: coral-red fluorescence of lesions.

Clues Sharp demarcation, light-brown color, fluorescence, site, demonstration of organism

Treatment Topically, 3% salicylic acid and 6% benzoic acid in O/W cream. Cleared in 3 weeks. Alternatives: oral erythromycin or topical imidazole cream.

XIII

Superficial

Fungal Infections

Dermatophyte Infections
Candidiasis
Tinea Versicolor

Dermatophyte Infections

GENERAL REMARKS

These are superficial infections caused by dermatophytes, i.e., fungi that thrive only in nonviable tissue of the skin or hair (stratum corneum, nails, hair). The three principal genera are *Microsporum, Trichophyton,* and *Epidermophyton;* they cause dermatophytosis, or *tinea* (used generically for dermatophytoses, e.g., tinea capitis).

EPIDEMIOLOGY AND ETIOLOGY

Age Children have scalp infections (*Microsporum* and *Trichophyton*) and young adults have intertriginous infections.

Sex No profound differences

Race Adult blacks are said to have a lower incidence of dermatophytosis.

Other Predisposing Factors *Immunosuppressed patients* have a higher incidence and more intractable dermatophytoses. With topical immunosuppression (i.e., with prolonged application of topical corticosteroids) there can be marked modification in the usual banal character of dermatophytosis; this is especially true of the face, groin, and hands.

HAIR

Epilated hairs should be studied immediately. Several hairs are placed on a slide, 10 or 20% potassium hydroxide and a coverslip are added, and the slide is warmed without boiling. After 15 to 30 min, the slide may be examined for the presence of fungi. For this and most other microscopic examinations, the substage or condenser diaphragm should be closed to approximately one-half its normal opening area and the condenser lowered until best contrast with the specimen is obtained.

SKIN SCRAPINGS (SCALES)

Several tiny pieces of the scrapings should be placed on a glass slide without overlapping. Potassium hydroxide (10 to 20%)[1]

and a coverslip are used; the specimen is gently heated and then allowed to stand for about 5 min. The specimen may then be studied for hyphae, arthrospores, or, occasionally, budding cells. One cannot identify specific organisms, usually, but only note their presence or absence.[2]

NAIL SCRAPINGS

Several thin pieces of the specimen should be placed on a glass slide without overlapping. A few drops of potassium hydroxide (10 to 20%) and a coverslip are used. The slide is gently heated to near-boiling and then allowed to sit for approximately *one-half hour.* Avoid boiling, which causes bubbles that both disrupt the fungus and produce artifacts. The specimen may then be studied for hyphae and budding cells.

---

[1] Specially prepared 2% KOH with ink and detergent (Swartz–Lamkins stain) may be used as an alternative to higher concentrations of KOH and is less likely to damage microscope lenses.

[2] Obtain fungal cultures for specific identification.

Tinea Pedis (Athlete's Foot)

ETIOLOGY

Predisposing Factors Hot, humid weather; occlusive footwear

PHYSICAL EXAMINATION

Skin Lesions

TYPE Scaling, plus maceration (Figure 72), and vesicles or bullae
COLOR Red; opaque white scales
DISTRIBUTION *Trichophyton mentagrophytes* localized between third and fourth interdigital spaces and later the sole, especially in the arch

LABORATORY AND SPECIAL EXAMINATIONS

Direct microscopic examination (see Figure 74) and culture
Trichophyton rubrum produces scaling and hyperkeratosis of the soles extending to the foot in the area covered by a ballet shoe (Figure 73)

TREATMENT

Acute Vesicular Stages Burow's wet dressings, followed by clotrimazole 1%

Subacute (Maceration, Scaling)

Cicloprox, clotrimazole cream or lotion, or miconazole
Liberal use of antifungal powders between the toes and in the shoes

Chronic

1. Same as treatment of Subacute
2. Whitfield's tincture (3% salicylic acid, 6% benzoic acid in 70% alcohol solution)
3. Griseofulvin, 500 mg orally bid with food for 3–6 months

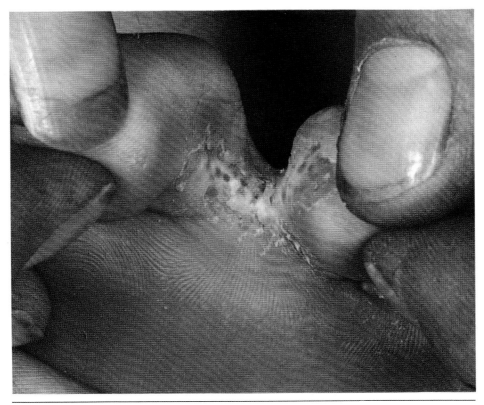

72 Tinea pedis interdigitalis (athlete's foot)

Patient Profile Twenty-three-year-old male

History For 2 months, skin lesions between toes III and IV of both feet

Physical Examination The interdigital spaces show maceration and scaling. In the groin, erythematosquamous patches with central healing.

Differential Diagnosis Erythrasma, interdigital psoriasis, intertrigo

Laboratory and Special Examinations Direct microscopic examination for fungi: septate and branched mycelia. Culture: Trichophyton rubrum. Scrapings from groin: same findings.

Clue Demonstration of fungi

Treatment Rapid clearing with miconazole cream for 4 weeks

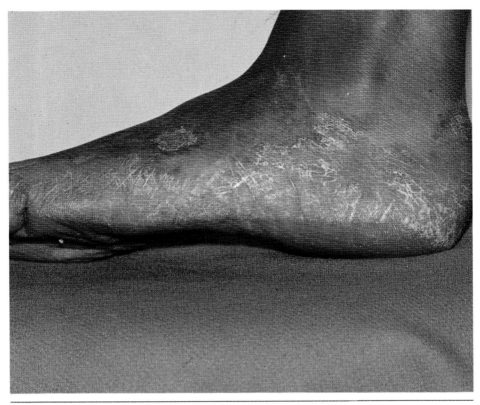

73 Tinea pedis

Patient Profile Thirty-two-year-old female

History For 10 years, nonpruritic, pink, scaling disorder of skin of feet

Physical Examination The soles, sides of the feet, and the heels show a faint pink color, covered with fine silvery-white scales. The upper border of these areas is irregular. Some of the nails are yellowish, thickened, and cracked.

Differential Diagnosis Hyperkeratosis, allergic contact dermatitis from shoes

Laboratory and Special Examinations Direct microscopic examination for fungi: septate and branched mycelia. Culture: Trichophyton rubrum.

Clues Pink discoloration with fine scaling, moccasin configuration, demonstration of fungi

Treatment Oral griseofulvin, 500 mg/day for 12 months. Topically, 5% salicylic acid and benzoic acid in O/W cream. Skin completely cleared; nails retained normal appearance. Recurrence of skin lesions within 5 months and nails within 1 year after cessation of therapy.

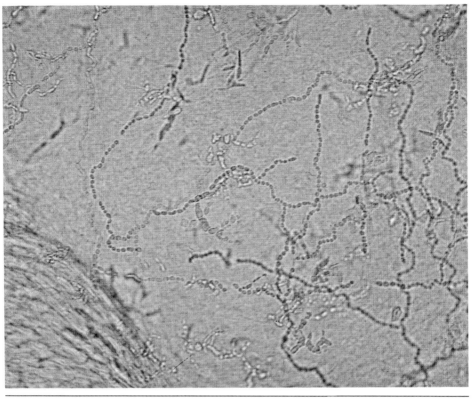

74   Trichophyton rubrum

Potassium hydroxide preparation of skin scrapings from patient in Figure 73. Septate and branched mycelia, indicative of pathogenic fungus

Tinea manus is a chronic dermatophytosis of the hand(s), often unilateral, and most commonly on the dominant hand, in which there is always a preexisting tinea pedis, usually toe and often fingernail dermatophytosis.

ETIOLOGY

Trichophyton rubrum

LABORATORY AND SPECIAL EXAMINATIONS

Direct microscopic examination of scales (see Figure 74) taken from the advancing crescentric edge

PHYSICAL EXAMINATION

Skin Lesions

TYPE   Hyperkeratosis, scaling vesicles in clusters
COLOR   Erythematous
SHAPE   Annular, polycyclic (see Figure 75), especially on the dorsum
DISTRIBUTION   Diffuse hyperkeratosis of the palms or patchy scaling on the dorsa and sides of fingers; 50 percent of patients have *unilateral* involvement

TREATMENT

Same as treatment outlined for chronic tinea pedis (see p. 196)

SIGNIFICANCE

Inasmuch as the nails may not respond to treatment or tinea manus may recur following treatment, this can be a frustrating problem and is especially difficult in patients who use their hands for fine skills or who are exposed to the public.

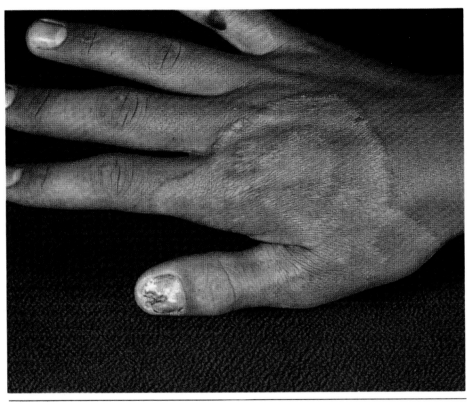

75 Tinea manus

Patient Profile Sixteen-year-old male

History For 3 months, a nonpruritic lesion on right hand and changes of thumb nail

Physical Examination On the dorsum of the hand, a large area that is less tanned than the surrounding skin and bordered by a narrow erythematous, slightly indurated delicate scaling zone. The margin is quite sharp and somewhat polycyclic. The thumb nail is cracked, discolored, and thickened (subungual keratosis). The other hand is not affected. Both feet also show erythematosquamous lesions.

Differential Diagnosis Granuloma annulare

Laboratory and Special Examinations Direct microscopic examination of skin and nail scrapings for fungi: septate and branched mycelia (see Figure 74). Culture: Trichophyton rubrum. Skin of feet: same findings.

Treatment Oral griseofulvin, 500 mg/day for 5 months. Topically, 5% salicylic acid and 10% benzoic acid in O/W cream. Skin of hands cleared in 2 months, the nails in 5 months.

Tinea cruris is a subacute or chronic dermatophytosis of the upper thigh in males, caused by *Epidermophyton floccosum* or *Trichophyton rubrum.*

EPIDEMIOLOGY AND ETIOLOGY

Age Young adults ("jock itch")
Sex Male
Predisposing Factors Warm, humid environment; tight clothing worn by men; obesity

HISTORY

Duration of Lesions Weeks, months
Skin Symptoms Pruritus, burning, paresthesia of the groin

PHYSICAL EXAMINATION

Skin Lesions

TYPE Plaques with scaling sharp margins with occasional pustules and central clearing
COLOR Dull red
ARRANGEMENT Arciform, polycyclic
DISTRIBUTION Intertriginous areas and adjacent upper thigh and buttock (Figure 76). Scrotum is rarely involved, in contrast to candidiasis

DIFFERENTIAL DIAGNOSIS

Wood's lamp examination is negative for coral-red fluorescence, as seen in erythrasma.

LABORATORY AND SPECIAL EXAMINATIONS

Direct microscopic examination of scrapings for mycelia (see Figure 74)

TREATMENT

For acute and subacute tinea cruris, use nonirritating lotions such as tolnaftate or miconazole.
If there is no response, or there is irritation from topical antifungals, then griseofulvin is indicated, 500 mg bid with food for 3 to 4 weeks.

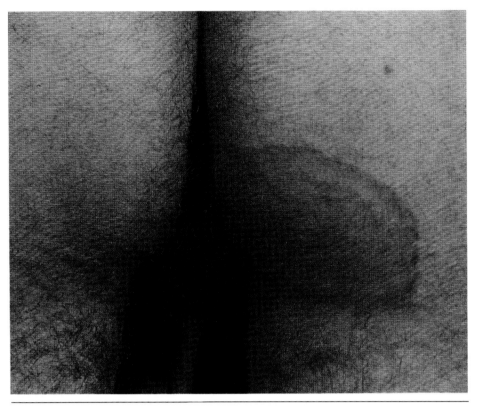

76 Tinea cruris

Patient Profile *Seventy-year-old male*

History *For 12 months, a nonpruritic lesion on right buttock, gradually extending. In addition, red scaling lesions on the soles and between the toes of the feet.*

Physical Examination *On the buttock is an 8 by 8 cm, round to ovoid, sharply demarcated area. The outer border consists of an erythematous, slightly elevated ring with barely perceptible fine scaling. The skin inside this ring has a somewhat normal appearance. Elsewhere there are two other incomplete rings and some less-well-defined erythematous spots.*

Laboratory and Special Examinations *Direct microscopic examination for fungi: positive (see Figure 74). Culture:* Trichophyton rubrum. *Skin scrapings from feet: same findings.*

Clues *Typical appearance and demonstration of fungi*

Treatment *Oral griseofulvin, 500 mg/day for 4 weeks. Topically, 5% salicylic acid and 5% benzoic acid in O/W cream. Lesion on buttock cleared in 4 weeks; skin of feet much improved but fungi still demonstrable.*

These scaling papular lesions occur in an annular arrangement with peripheral enlargement and central clearing on the trunk, limbs, or face.

EPIDEMIOLOGY AND ETIOLOGY

Age All ages
Occupation Animal (large and small) workers
Predisposing Factors Infection is acquired from an active lesion of an animal, by direct human contact *(Trichophyton rubrum),* or, rarely, from soil.

PHYSICAL EXAMINATION

Skin Lesions

TYPE Small to large, scaling, sharply marginated plaques with or without pustules or vesicles (Figure 77)
SHAPE AND ARRANGEMENT Peripheral enlargement and central clearing, producing an annular configuration
DISTRIBUTION Single and occasionally scattered multiple lesions
SITES OF PREDILECTION Exposed skin of forearm, neck

DIFFERENTIAL DIAGNOSIS

Tinea faciale, especially in patients with AIDS

LABORATORY AND SPECIAL EXAMINATIONS

Direct microscopic examination of scales from the advancing border, prepared with 10% potassium hydroxide

TREATMENT

Topical antifungal creams (2% micronazole cream) bid for 7 to 10 days. If extensive or resistant to topical treatment, griseofulvin is indicated, combined with topical antifungal preparations.

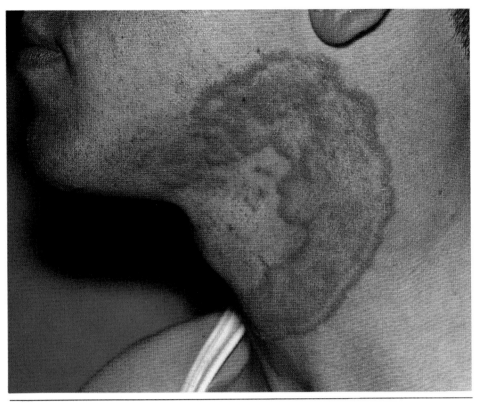

77 Tinea corporis

Patient Profile Twenty-three-year-old male

History For 4 months, red lesion on neck, gradually extending. Interdigital webs of toes show scaling. No pruritus.

Physical Examination On left side of neck, large half-moon-shaped lesion. The border is red, irregular, and somewhat polycyclic, about 4 mm broad, slightly elevated, the upper parts showing a delicate scaling. The skin between the borders is, in part, normal and shows elsewhere erythematous macules and papules.

Laboratory and Special Examinations Direct microscopic examination for fungi: septate and branched mycelia. Culture: Trichophyton rubrum. Interdigital webs of feet: same findings.

Clues Typical appearance, demonstration of fungi

Treatment Oral griseofulvin 500 mg/day for 4 weeks, miconazole cream topically

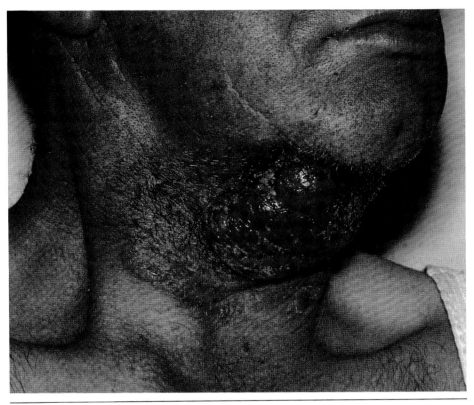

78 Tinea barbae (kerion-like)

Patient Profile *Forty-nine-year-old stock farmer*

History *For 14 days, boil-like painless tumors under the chin. No fever. Some of his cows show scaling patches.*

Physical Examination *In the bearded area under the chin is a sharply demarcated red nodule, 4 × 6 cm, composed of several confluent lobular infiltrates. The surface is moist and partly covered with crusts. On many sites pus exudes from the nodules. Beard hairs near the border and their roots are enveloped with a whitish cuff. The surrounding part of the nodule shows red scaling areas. Regional lymph nodes are not enlarged.*

Differential Diagnosis *Carbuncle, malignant lymphoma, sporotrichosis, actinomycosis, nocardiosis*

Laboratory and Special Examinations *Direct microscopic examination for fungi on loose beard hairs: septate and branched mycelia.* Culture: Trichophyton verrucosum. *Bacterial culture:* Staphylococcus aureus *hemolytica.*

Clues *Site of the lesions, occupation, demonstration of fungus*

Treatment *Oral griseofulvin, 500 mg/day for 2 months. Topically, 10% salicylic acid and 10% sulfur in O/W cream. In addition, oral penicillin for 2 weeks. Clearing in 6 weeks*

This subacute or chronic dermatophytosis produces scaly patches of scalp alopecia, or sometimes scarring alopecia, and largely affects children.

EPIDEMIOLOGY AND ETIOLOGY

Age Children or, rarely, adults
Pathogenesis Invasion of hair shaft by the dermatophytes, principally *Microsporum audouini* (child to child, via barber, hats, theatre seats) and *M. canis* (young pets to child and then child to child)

HISTORY

Duration of Lesions Weeks to months
Skin Symptoms Loss of hair; pain and tenderness in inflammatory type

PHYSICAL EXAMINATION

Skin Lesions and Hair Changes

FOUR TYPES

"*Gray patch*" *ringworm* Brittle hair; shafts break off close to scalp surface. Caused by *M. audouini* and *M. canis* (see Figure 79)
"*Black dot*" *ringworm* Broken-off hairs near surface give appearance of "dots." Tends to be diffuse and poorly circumscribed. Caused by

Trichophyton tonsurans and *T. violaceum*
"*Kerion*" *(Greek, "honeycomb")* Boggy, elevated, purulent, inflamed nodule (see Figure 78)
Favus See Figure 80.

LABORATORY AND SPECIAL EXAMINATIONS

Fluorescence Examination with Wood's Lamp Examination of scalp with filtered ultraviolet (Wood's light) reveals bright green hair shafts in scalp infections caused by *M. audouini* and *M. canis*. *T. schoenleini* fluorescence is grayish green.
Direct Microscopic Examination with 10% Potassium Hydroxide Spores can be seen surrounding the hair shaft (*T. tonsurans* and *T. violaceum*).

TREATMENT

Griseofulvin: (1) "gray patch" ringworm, 250 mg bid for 1 or 2 months (or 5 mg/kg for children); (2) "black dot" ringworm, longer treatment and higher doses—continued 2 weeks after Wood's lamp, potassium hydroxide, and cultures are negative.

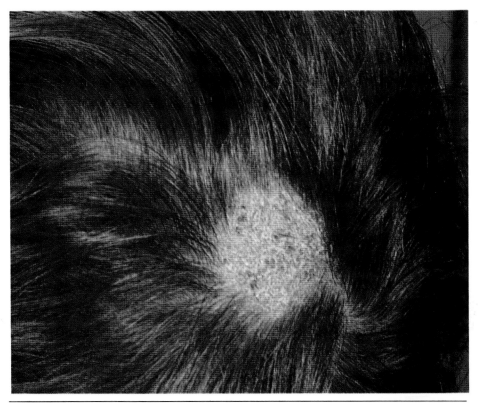

79 Tinea capitis from Microsporum canis

Patient Profile Four-year-old boy

History For 2 months, nonpruritic, round, white scaling lesions on scalp, associated with hair loss. Five cats had had scaling bald spots which cleared spontaneously.

Physical Examination On the scalp is an erythematous, somewhat sharply demarcated round area, 3 cm in diameter, with diffuse delicate white scaling and nearly complete loss of hair.

Laboratory and Special Examinations Direct microscopic examination for fungi of scales and hairs: mycelia. Culture: Microsporum canis. Wood's light examination of hair: green fluorescence.

Clues Scaling alopecia, demonstration of fungus

Treatment Oral griseofulvin, 250 mg/day for 4 months. Topically, 5% salicylic acid and 10% benzoic acid in O/W cream. Completely healed, including hair growth, in 6 months.

Tinea Capitis (Favus)

Cutaneous atrophy, scar formation, and baldness are typical of favus, due to infection with *Trichophyton schoenleini.* So-called scutula, i.e., yellowish adherent crusts, are present on the scalp. Only in the marginal zones does the hair still grow normally. Favus (Latin, "honeycomb") has now become very uncommon in Western Europe. In some parts of the world (Middle East, South Africa), however, it is still endemic.

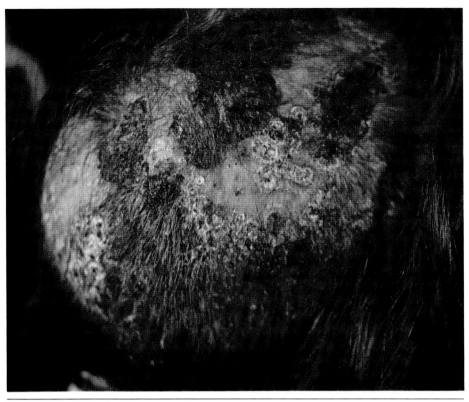

80 *Tinea capitis from* Trichophyton schoenleini *(favus)*

Patient Profile *Fifty-five-year-old female, mentally retarded*

History *Since childhood, loss of hair and crusts on scalp. Wears a wig and until recently refused any treatment.*

Physical Examination *Extensive bald areas on scalp with hypopigmentation, atrophy, and absence of follicles. In addition, thick yellowish squamous crusts (scutula) and some erosive areas, particularly along the borders.*

Differential Diagnosis *Tinea capitis from* Trichophyton violaceum *or* Microsporum canis

Laboratory and Special Examinations *Direct microscopic examination of loose hairs for fungi: septate and branched mycelia. Culture:* Trichophyton schoenleini. *Wood's light: hairs fluoresce blue-green. Bacterial culture: negative.*

Clues *Irreversible scarring alopecia, yellow crusts, demonstration of fungi*

Treatment *Oral griseofulvin, 500 mg/day for 6 months. Topically, 5% salicylic acid and 10% benzoic acid in O/W cream. Cleared in 5 months, except for irreversible alopecia.*

Significance *In highly civilized countries extremely rare nowadays. Does not heal spontaneously after puberty and is contagious, especially to children.*

Candidiasis (Moniliasis)

Candidiasis is caused by *Candida albicans,* which produces a variety of lesions on skin and mucous membranes.

EPIDEMIOLOGY AND ETIOLOGY

Age Infants (diaper area, mouth), any age

Sex Women (vulvovaginitis with diabetes), males (balanitis)

Occupation Persons who immerse their hands in water; housewives; bartenders; florists; HIV-infected individuals with prolonged use of steroid inhalants; bakers develop paronychia

Other Predisposing Factors Diabetes, obesity, hyperhidrosis, heat, maceration, immunologic defects (depressed T-cell function), polyendocrinopathies, pregnancy, oral contraceptives, systemic antibacterial agents, systemic and topical corticosteroids, chronic debilitation (carcinoma, leukemia), chemotherapy

COMMON CLINICAL TYPES (See Figure XIV.)

Vulvovaginitis Pruritus; thick creamy-white, curdy discharge; meaty red erythema of vaginal skin and mucous membrane. Spreads to perineum and groin. Satellite pustules.

Balanitis See Figure 84.

Oral Candidiasis ("Thrush") Creamy-white areas of membranous exudate on

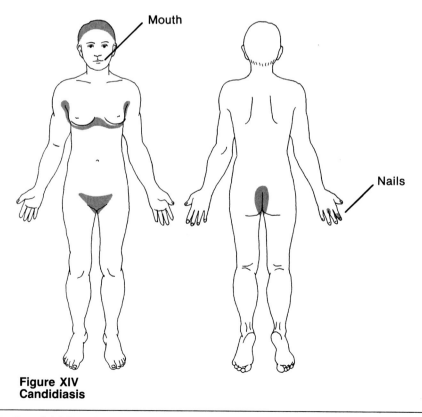

Figure XIV
Candidiasis

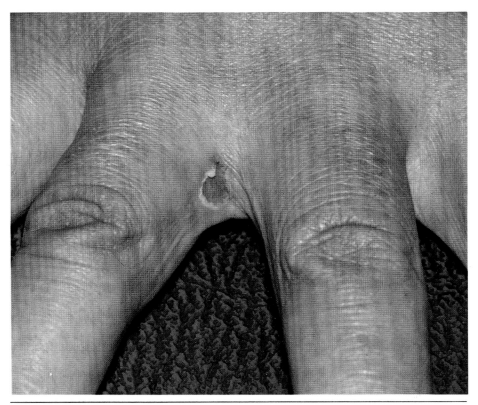

81 Candidiasis (interdigital)

Patient Profile Forty-three-year-old nurse

History For 4 weeks, small erosive and scaling lesion on third interdigital web of right hand

Physical Examination Round to ovoid erosion, surrounded by a delicate cigarette-paper-like scaling collar (collarette)

Laboratory and Special Examinations Direct microscopic examination for fungi and yeasts: Candida *(see Figure 86)*. Culture: Candida albicans.

Clues Location, scaling collar, demonstration of Candida

Treatment Nystatin ointment. Clearing required 3 months. Prevention: keeping the interdigital web as dry as possible.

the tongue or buccal mucosa that can be easily removed. *Perlèche* occurs at the corners of the mouth and is characterized by painful fissures and erosions.

Diaper Candidiasis See Figure 85.

Interdigital and Intertriginous Candidiasis See Figures 81 and 82, respectively.

Paronychial Candidiasis See Figure 83.

Follicular Candidiasis

LABORATORY AND SPECIAL EXAMINATIONS

Direct microscopic examination of crusts or scales using Gram's stain or 5% potassium hydroxide preparation (see Figure 86). Culture is essential for identification of *C. albicans.*

TREATMENT

Vulvovaginitis
Vaginal tablets or suppositories used once daily at bedtime (for 3–7 nights): clotrimizole, miconazole

Male partners should also be treated to prevent conjugal candidiasis

Balanitis Imidazole cream followed by nystatin powder. Keep foreskin retracted.

Oral Candidiasis (Thrush'') Nystatin suspension. Clotrimazole troches qid for 3 weeks. One percent gentian violet (aqueous) is highly effective but stains the mouth.

Diaper Candidiasis Topical nystatin ointment plus liberal use of powder. Avoid rubber or plastic diaper pants.

Interdigital and Intertriginous Candidiasis For interdigital involvement, use nystatin cream. For intertriginous involvement, air-dry frequently; loose clothing; topical nystatin ointment followed by nystatin powder or miconazole; oral ketoconazole. Castellani's paint is very effective.

Paronychial Candidiasis Application of gentian violet in water, 2%, deeply under nail fold once daily. Eliminate immersion in water. Topical miconazole. Oral ketoconazole is sometimes indicated if gentian violet fails.

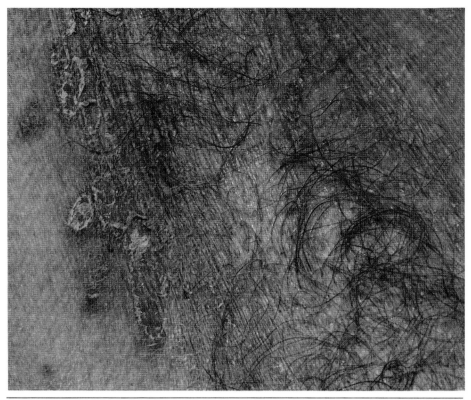

82 Candidiasis (intertriginous)

Patient Profile Fifty-nine-year-old male

History For 6 weeks, "eczematous" lesions in right groin, occasionally pruritic

Physical Examination In right groin, a nonindurated, fairly sharp but irregularly demarcated erythematous area with easily detachable cigarette-paper-like scaling that follows the borders of the lesion, occasionally circular, resulting in a scaling collar. Outside the main lesion are some smaller similar lesions (satellites).

Differential Diagnosis Seborrheic dermatitis, psoriasis

Laboratory and Special Examinations Potassium hydroxide preparation of skin scrapings: Candida *(see Figure 86)*. Culture: Candida albicans. No diabetes present.

Clues Erythematous area with scaling collar, satellites, demonstration of C. albicans

Treatment Miconazole cream. Cleared in 3 weeks.

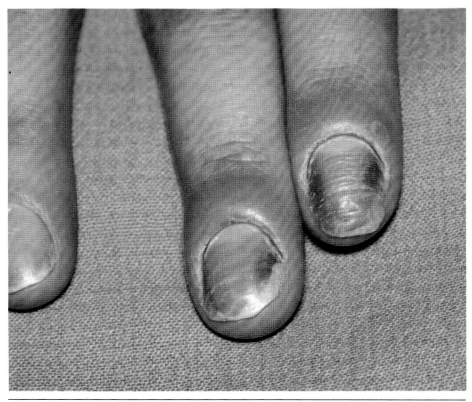

83 Onychia and paronychia from Candida albicans

Patient Profile Sixteen-year-old female housecleaner

History For 1 year, red swelling of the skin around nails IV and V of left hand. Painful on pressure.

Physical Examination Redness and swelling of the nail folds. The eponychia are absent. The sides of the nails are yellowish-gray and show distal onycholysis and an irregular surface.

Differential Diagnosis Paronychia and onychia from Candida albicans, bacterial paronychia with secondary nail changes, onychia from Trichophyton rubrum

Laboratory and Special Examinations Potassium hydroxide preparation of skin and nail scrapings: pseudomycelia and clusters of yeast cells (see Figure 86). Culture: C. albicans. Immunologic screening, including neutrophil phagocytosis and killing: not impaired. No diabetes present.

Treatment Nystatin ointment, subsequently miconazole cream with and without occlusive plastic dressing. Much improved in 3 months. Patient has to avoid getting skin wet and should not remove the eponychia.

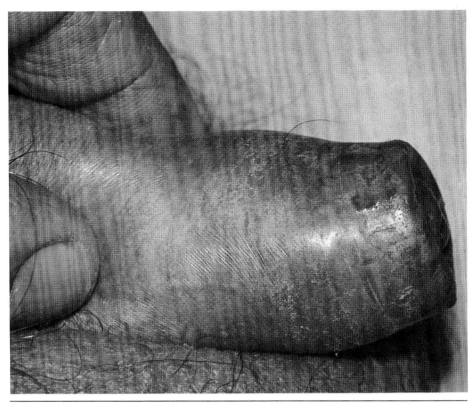

84 Candidiasis of the penis (balanoposthitis from Candida albicans)

Patient Profile Fifty-two-year-old male

History For 6 weeks, painful, erosive and scaling lesions with slight edema of preputium and glans penis. For 10 years, diabetes mellitus, recently uncontrolled. No sexual intercourse.

Physical Examination Preputium shows linear erosions, slight edema, erythema, and delicate scaling. Erosive areas on glans penis.

Clues Linear erosions (fissures) on preputium, delicate scaling, demonstration of C. albicans

Laboratory and Special Examinations Direct microscopic examination for yeasts: Candida (see Figure 86). Culture: C. albicans. Diabetes present.

Treatment Nystatin ointment and control of diabetes. Cleared in 3 weeks. Alternatives: miconazole or clotrimazole.

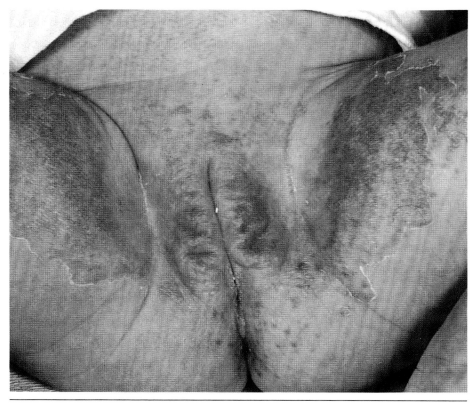

85 Candidiasis of the groin in an infant

Patient Profile Four-month-old girl

History For 3 weeks, red scaling lesions on vulva and inner sides of thighs

Physical Examination Red macular lesions on vulva and in groin. On the inner sides of the thighs are large red areas, not sharply demarcated, in part denuded, and surrounded by a delicate scaling collar (collarette). Outside the main lesions are a few satellite lesions.

Differential Diagnosis Diaper dermatitis, seborrheic dermatitis

Laboratory and Special Examinations Direct examination for yeasts: mycelial pseudomycelia and yeast cells (see Figure 86). Culture: C. albicans. No evidence of diabetes.

Clues Scaling collar, satellite lesions, demonstration of Candida

Treatment Nystatin ointment with 1% hydrocortisone. Cleared in 3 weeks. Frequent changes of diaper, avoidance of plastic pants.

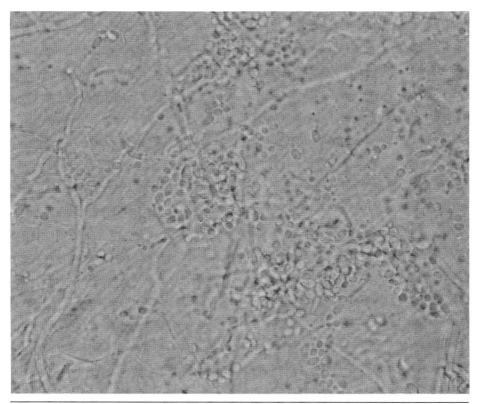

86 Candida *in potassium hydroxide preparation: pseudomycelia and clusters of grapelike yeast cells*

Tinea Versicolor (Pityriasis Versicolor)

This is a chronic asymptomatic fungous infection of the trunk and is characterized by white or brown macules and caused by *Pityrosporum orbiculare.*

EPIDEMIOLOGY AND ETIOLOGY

Age Young adults
Predisposing Factors Climatic factors appear to be important as the disease is far more common in the tropics and in the summer in temperate climates. High levels of cortisol appear to increase susceptibility—both in Cushing's syndrome and with prolonged administration of corticosteroids.

HISTORY

Duration of Lesions Months to years
Skin Symptoms None

PHYSICAL EXAMINATION

Skin Lesions

TYPE Macule, sharply marginated, with fine scaling that is easily scraped off with the edge of a glass microscopic slide
COLOR Brown of varying intensities and hues (Figure 87); "off white" macules (Figure 88)
SIZE AND SHAPE Round or oval macules varying in size from 1.0 cm to very large areas (>30.0 cm)
DISTRIBUTION Scattered discrete lesions
SITES OF PREDILECTION Upper trunk (Figure 87), upper arms, neck, abdomen, axillae, groin, thighs, genitalia. Rarely on the face

DIFFERENTIAL DIAGNOSIS

Tinea versicolor is recognized by the distribution and shape of the lesions and is eas-ily identified by examination of the scales for fungus. The hypopigmented type may be confused with vitiligo, but careful examination of all the lesions with Wood's lamp reveals scales with a pale yellow-green fluorescence, and these will contain the fungus.

LABORATORY AND SPECIAL EXAMINATIONS

Direct Microscopic Examination of Scales Prepared with Potassium Hydroxide Hyphae and spores referred to as "spaghetti and meat balls"
Wood's Lamp Examination Faint yellow-green fluorescence of scales

PATHOPHYSIOLOGY

Dicarboxylic acids formed by enzymatic oxidation of fatty acids in skin surface lipids inhibit tyrosinase in epidermal melanocytes and thereby lead to hypomelanosis. The enzyme is present in the organism.

TREATMENT

Scrubbing off scales with soap and water
Short applications of selenium sulfide (2%) for 12 nights, wash off in 30 minutes. Repeat every 2 weeks.
Miconazole cream
Topical ketoconazole (2%)
When frequent recurrences: short course (e.g., 3 weeks) of oral ketoconazole, 200 mg daily

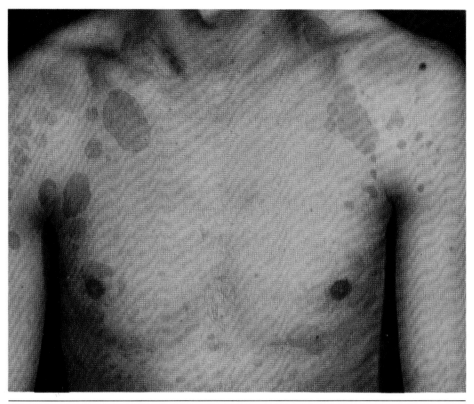

87 Tinea versicolor (pityriasis versicolor)

Patient Profile *Twenty-four-year-old male*

History *For 2 years, nonpruritic eruption of light brown spots on trunk*

Physical Examination *On and around the shoulders, several light brown macules with sharp margins varying in size from 0.5 to 5.0 cm; delicate scaling perceptible after scratching. A few similar lesions on the chest.*

Differential Diagnosis *Seborrheic dermatitis*

Laboratory and Special Examinations *Direct microscopic examination for fungi and yeasts: short, stout hyphal elements and clusters of rounded budding spores.*

Clues *Clinical appearance, scaling after scratching, location, demonstration of organisms*

Treatment *Cleared in 3 weeks with 3% salicylic acid and 6% benzoic acid in O/W cream. Alternatives: selenium sulfide topically or an imidazole cream.*

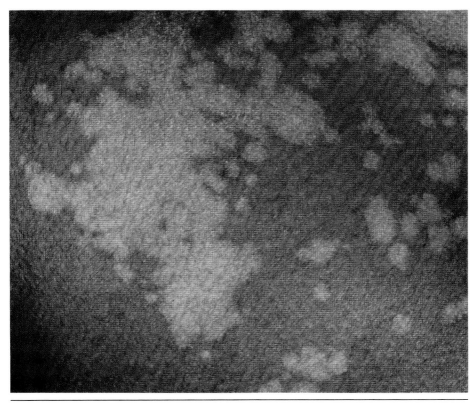

88   Tinea versicolor with hypomelanosis (pityriasis versicolor alba)

Patient Profile   Twenty-nine-year-old Caucasian male

History   For 3 months, nonpruritic white spots on trunk

Physical Examination   On the upper part of the back and the chest are numerous sharply demarcated, round or ovoid depigmented macules, varying in size from 0.5 to 4.0 cm, partly merging. On gentle scratching with the nail, a delicate scaling is perceptible. The nonaffected skin is tanned. Patient has Skin Type III.

Differential Diagnosis   Vitiligo, hypomelanosis secondary to other disorders, e.g., pinta, leprosy, cleared psoriasis, nummular eczema, etc.

Laboratory and Special Examinations   Direct microscopic examination for fungi and yeasts (see Figure 74)

Clues   Location, delicate scaling, demonstration of organisms

Treatment   Topically, 5% salicylic acid and 5% benzoic acid in O/W cream. Alternatives: selenium sulfide or an imidazole cream.

XIV

Viral Skin

Infections

Verruca Vulgaris (Common Wart)

This discrete benign epithelial hyperplasia is manifested as papules and plaques caused by the human wart virus of the papova group, human papilloma virus (HPV) 1, 2, 3.

HISTORY

Duration of Lesions Weeks, months
Skin Symptoms None, except on palms and soles, where pain and tenderness can occur

Verruca Vulgaris
(See Figure 89)

EPIDEMIOLOGY AND ETIOLOGY

Age School children; incidence decreases after age 25
Sex Girls more than boys
Other Factors Contagion occurs in groups—small (home) or large (school gymnasium). Verruca vulgaris and condyloma accuminatum viruses are antigenically distinct. Verruca vulgaris, however, rarely occurs on the penile shaft. More common and widespread in immunosuppressed patients.

PHYSICAL EXAMINATION

Skin Lesions

TYPE Firm papules, 1 to 10 mm or rarely larger, hyperkeratotic surface, with vegetations
COLOR Skin color, characteristic *"red dots" (thrombosing capillary loops)* seen with hand lens (Figure 89, look at 11 to 12 o'clock position)
SHAPE Round
ARRANGEMENT Isolated lesion, scattered discrete lesions
SITES OF PREDILECTION Sites of trauma—hands, fingers, knees

DIFFERENTIAL DIAGNOSIS

The red dots (thrombosed capillary loops) as a diagnostic marker have not been emphasized—these are pathognomonic and best seen with a 7X to 10X hand lens after application of a drop of mineral oil.

TREATMENT

For small lesions: salicylic acid and lactic acid in collodion

For large lesions: 40% salicylic acid plaster for 1 week, then application of salicylic acid–lactic acid in collodion
Liquid nitrogen (10–30 seconds) or electrocautery, but never surgery
Laser surgery

Verruca Plantaris

EPIDEMIOLOGY AND ETIOLOGY

Age Five to twenty-five, but can occur at any age
Sex Females more than males
Other Factors Trauma is a factor as the lesions often occur on sites of pressure.
Etiology Human papilloma virus (HPV) 1, 2, and 3

PHYSICAL EXAMINATION

Skin Lesions

TYPE Early small, shiny, sharply marginated papule → plaque with rough hyperkeratotic surface, often covered by a callus-like hyperkeratosis
COLOR Skin-colored. To identify diagnostic red dots, many plantar warts must be pared with a scalpel to remove the overlying hyperkeratosis.
PALPATION Tenderness may be marked, especially in certain acute types
DISTRIBUTION

Extent Usually one but may be three to six or more
Sites Pressure points, heads of metatarsal, heels, toes

TREATMENT

If asymptomatic, no treatment, as 50 percent disappear in 6 months
Do not excise (recur with painful scars)
Do not use electrocautery (recur with scars)
Forty percent salicylic acid plaster for 1 week, then liquid nitrogen or salicylic acid–lactic acid in collodion

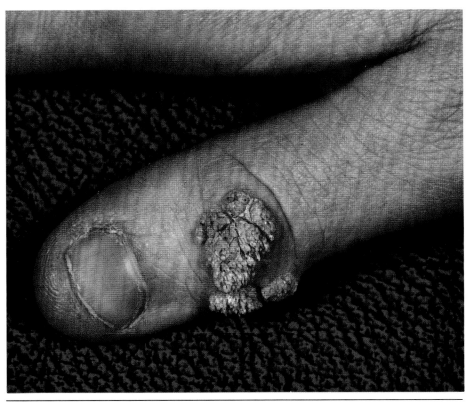

89 Verruca vulgaris (common wart)

Patient Profile Twenty-two-year-old female homemaker

History For several years, warts which had been treated previously elsewhere

Physical Examination Three lesions 0.5 to 1.5 cm in diameter with a filiform surface, on the right thumb

Treatment Application of liquid nitrogen. After four applications at 3-week intervals, the warts disappeared.

Relieve pressure with metatarsal bar (on the outside of the shoes)
Laser surgery
Hyperthermia using hot water (113°F)

immersion for 1/2 to 3/4 hour 2 or 3 times weekly for 16 treatments is often effective, as the wart virus is thermolabile.

Verruca Plana ("Flat Wart")

EPIDEMIOLOGY AND ETIOLOGY

Age Young children of both sexes
Sex Women under 20
Etiology Human papilloma virus (HPV) 1, 2, 3, 10, and 11

PHYSICAL EXAMINATION

Skin Lesions

TYPE Papules (1 to 5 mm), "flat" surface without a "wartily fissured" surface; the thickness of the lesion is 1 to 2 mm (Figure 90)
COLOR Skin-colored or light brown
SHAPE Round, oval, polygonal, linear lesions (Koebner's or isomorphic phenomenon: induction of lesions by physical trauma)
DISTRIBUTION Always numerous discrete lesions, closely set
SITES OF PREDILECTION Face, dorsa of hands, shins

TREATMENT

Avoid drastic destructive treatments as the lesions tend to spontaneously disappear, often after suggestion alone.
Retinoic acid cream, 0.1%, once daily, may be tried.

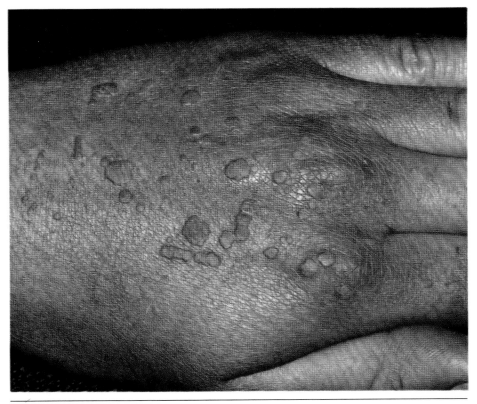

90 Verruca plana

Patient Profile Eight-year-old boy

History For 3 months, flat lesions on the back of the left hand

Physical Examination Round, firm, flat, rose-colored papules, some in linear arrangement, ranging in size from 1 to 4 mm in diameter, disseminated over the back of the left hand

Clue Typical clinical morphology (see Physical Examination)

Treatment Application of liquid nitrogen. After a number of treatments the lesions disappeared.

Condyloma Acuminatum (Genital Wart)

These soft, skin-colored, fleshy warts resemble a cauliflower and are caused by the human papilloma virus (HPV) of the papova group (HPV 6, 11, 16, 18, 31, 33).

EPIDEMIOLOGY AND ETIOLOGY

Age   Young adults, infants, and children
Etiology   The virus is immunologically distinct from the verruca vulgaris virus.
Transmission   Highly contagious, non-sexually and sexually transmitted. Ninety to 100 percent of partners of infected females are HPV infected.
Incubation Period   4–6 weeks

HISTORY

Duration of Lesions   Months to years
Skin Symptoms   Usually asymptomatic

PHYSICAL EXAMINATION

Skin Lesions

TYPE   Pin-head papules or cauliflower-like masses (see Figure 91)
COLOR   Skin colored, pink, or red
PALPATION   soft
SHAPE   Filliform, sessile (especially on penis) (see Figure 91)
DISTRIBUTION   Rarely few isolated lesions, usually in clusters
SITES OF PREDILECTION
Male   Frenulum, corona, glans, prepuce, meatus, shaft, scrotum
Female   Labia, clitoris, periurethral area, perineum, vagina, cervix (flat lesions)
Both sexes   Perianal area

LABORATORY AND SPECIAL EXAMINATIONS

Acetowhitening: Subclinical lesions can be visualized by wrapping the penis with gauze soaked with 5% acetic acid for 5 minutes. Using a 10× hand lens or culposcope, warts appear as tiny white papules.
Serologic test for syphilis: Negative

DIFFERENTIAL DIAGNOSIS

Condylomata lata—these are lesions of secondary syphilis and may be the only skin manifestation. They are flat (Latin *lata,* "flat"), not papillomatous, have a broad base, and are also strongly darkfield positive, with positive STS. All patients with condylomata acuminata should have an STS. *Lichen planus, normal sebaceous glands.*

COURSE AND PROGNOSIS

HPV types 16, 18, 31, and 33 are the major etiologic factors for cervical dysplasia and cervical squamous cell carcinoma; bowenoid papuloses in situ and invasive carcinoma of both the vulva and penis; anal squamous cell carcinoma of homosexual/bisexual males. Children delivered vaginally of mothers with genital HPV infection are at risk for developing recurrent respiratory papillomatosis in later life.

TREATMENT AND MANAGEMENT

Podophyllin, 25%, in tincture of benzoin, applied once weekly. Allow to dry and cover with talcum powder. The area should be washed off in 6 to 8 hr after each treatment. (Do not use during pregnancy.) Giant lesions around the anus (males) and in the vulva may require surgery.
Trichloracetic acid for flat lesions on penile shaft or glans, and labia.
Liquid nitrogen.
Electrocautery under local anesthesia.
Laser treatment very effective.
Intralesional injection of interferon.

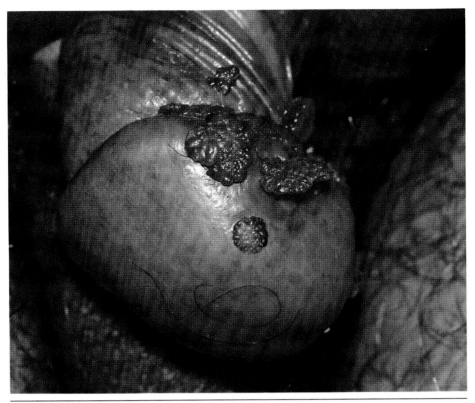

91 Condyloma acuminatum

Patient Profile Twenty-six-year-old bricklayer

History For 1 year, an excrescence on the penis

Physical Examination Soft, elongated, in part filiform tumor mass on the glans penis and preputium

Laboratory and Special Examinations Serologic test for syphilis: negative.

Clues Clinical morphology, absence of serologic evidence of syphilis

Treatment After a few applications of 25% podophyllin in ethanol the excrescences disappeared.

Molluscum Contagiosum

These discrete, umbilicated, pearly-white papules are caused by a poxvirus and occur in children and adults.

EPIDEMIOLOGY

Age Children (may be epidemic); adults (often sexually transmitted)
Sex Males more than females
Risk Factors HIV-infected individuals may have hundreds of small mollusca or giant mollusca on the face

HISTORY

Duration of Lesions Develop in 2 to 3 months
Skin Symptoms None, rarely pruritic if secondarily infected

PHYSICAL EXAMINATION

Skin Lesions

TYPE Papules (1 to 2 mm), nodules (5 to 10 mm) (rarely giant) (see Figure 93)
COLOR Pearly-white or skin-colored
SHAPE Round, oval, hemispherical, umbilicated (see Figure 92)
DISTRIBUTION Isolated single lesion or multiple scattered discrete lesions

SITES OF PREDILECTION Neck, trunk, anogenital area, eyelids

DIFFERENTIAL DIAGNOSIS

Keratoacanthoma (central keratotic plug); *basal cell carcinoma* (hard, telangiectasia). In HIV-infected individuals, cutaneous dissemination of *Histoplasma capsulatum* or *Cryptococcus neoformans* may be present with molluscum-like facial papules.

LABORATORY EXAMINATION

Direct microscopic examination of Giemsa-stained central semisolid core (obtained by pointed scalpel without local anesthesia) reveals "molluscum bodies" (inclusion bodies).

TREATMENT

Liquid nitrogen (10–15 seconds)
Light electrocautery

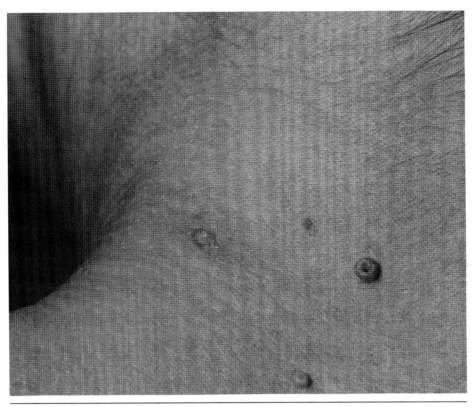

92 Molluscum contagiosum

Patient Profile Twenty-five-year-old male carpenter

History For 3 months, "tumors" on the neck

Physical Examination Three pale isolated umbilicated papules on the neck with a central umbilicus

Differential Diagnosis Fibromata, nevi

Laboratory and Special Examinations A core could be expressed from the lesions. Identification of molluscum bodies (virus-transformed epithelial cells).

Clues Typical clinical morphology and expression of curdlike core. Verification of contents by smear.

Pathophysiology Interaction of a specific DNA virus and epidermal cells

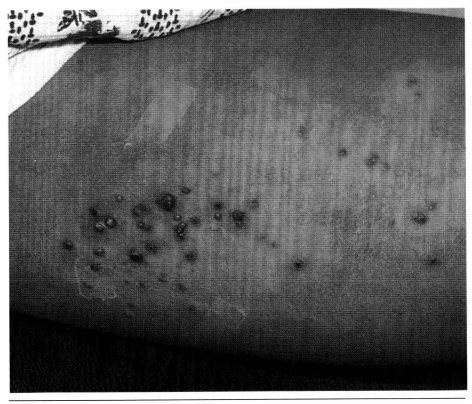

93 Molluscum contagiosum

Patient Profile Fourteen-year-old girl

History For 3 months, gradually increasing number of papules on the left shoulder, breast, and neck

Physical Examination On the left shoulder, irregularly disseminated, pinpoint to pinhead red papules, a number of them with a yellow top, a few with central umbilication

Laboratory and Special Examinations On pressure, a yellow curdlike core is expressed

Clues Clinical morphology and expression of core

Treatment Curettage after freezing with ethyl chloride

Herpes Simplex

Herpes simplex is an acute vesicular eruption on the skin and mucous membrane caused by *Herpesvirus hominis,* or herpes simplex virus (Types I and II) or HSV 1 and HSV 2.

EPIDEMIOLOGY AND ETIOLOGY

Age Primary infection in ages 1 to 5 years; in adults primary infection is acquired by mouth or genital contact

Occupation Medical personnel doing intensive care develop herpes infections of the finger (herpetic whitlow)

Other Factors Ultraviolet radiation, immunosuppression

Transmission Asymptomatic "carriers" may "shed" the virus and may transmit the disease. In general, HSV 1 infections are oral-labial and HSV 2 infections are genital. Genital herpes and oral-labial HSV infections can be caused by either HSV 1 or HSV 2. Transmission of HSV through genital intercourse occurs more frequently among persons with HSV 2. Furthermore, the frequency of clinical recurrence of genital infection is higher in persons with HSV 2 infections.

Incubation Period: Two to 20 days

Type I Herpes Simplex

PRIMARY INFECTION

Age One to five years and young adults

Skin Symptoms Tingling, burning and itching

Constitutional Symptoms Headache, fever

Skin Lesions

TYPE Pinhead size; vesicles on an erythematous base then erosions, crusts

ARRANGEMENT Herpetiform (in clusters)

SITES OF PREDILECTION Mouth (tongue, palate, buccal mucosa, gums with gingivostomatitis) *in primary infections only*

Lymphadenopathy Regional lymph nodes enlarged and tender

RECURRENT

Incidence One percent of population, and is a more difficult problem than the primary infection

Age Incidence increases rapidly after age 15 until age 30

Skin Lesions

TYPE Red edematous papule → small group of vesicles (see Figures 94 and 95)

ARRANGEMENT Herpetiform, linear, zosteriform (see Figure 94)

DISTRIBUTION Face, lips, or anywhere. *Only rarely* lesions occur on the mucous membrane

Miscellaneous Neurologic pain may precede each recurrence by 1 or 2 days. Mimics herpes zoster. Erythema multiforme may occur in 3 to 4 days or longer after a recurrence of herpes simplex

PATHOPHYSIOLOGY

The virus remains in the ganglion and may be reactivated related to sunlight, fever.

LABORATORY DIAGNOSIS

Tzanck Preparation Unroof the blister top carefully and gently scrape the floor and smear and air dry. Giemsa stain reveals multinucleate giant epithelial cells.

Culture of Virus Material from early vesicles is readily grown in tissue culture—grows rapidly (1 to 3 days)

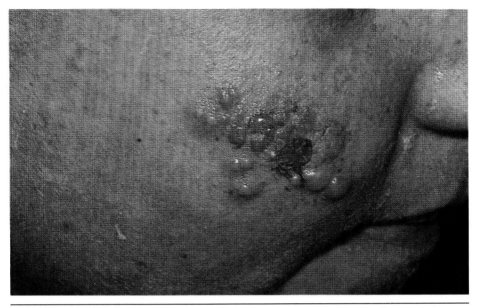

94a   Herpes simplex, recurrent

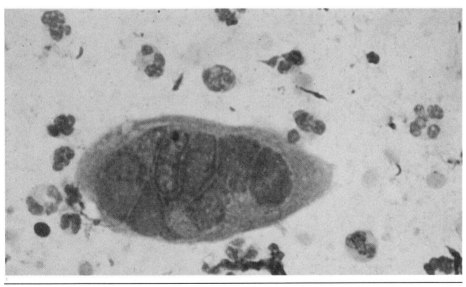

94b   Tzanck preparation showing multinucleate giant epithelial cell (Giemsa stain)
(Courtesy of Dr. Arthur R. Rhodes)

Patient Profile   *Five-year-old boy*

History   *Since early childhood, with intervals of varying length, an eruption on the right cheek*

Physical Examination   *In a serpiginous demarcated area 3 × 1.5 cm, primarily vesicles with clear and turbid content, sequential crusts*

Differential Diagnosis   *Impetigo, eczema*

Laboratory and Special Examinations   *For virus: Herpesvirus hominis type 1. For bacteria: no bacterial growth.*

VULVOVAGINITIS: PRIMARY

Constitutional Symptoms Fever, malaise
Skin Symptoms Pain, dysuria

Skin Lesions

TYPE

Vesicles → erosions → gray-white ulcerations
Edematous vulvar thickening
ARRANGEMENT Herpetiform (grouped vesicles and erosions)
SITES OF PREDILECTION Vaginal mucosa, cervix, labia, clitoris, perineum
Lymphadenopathy Tender regional lymphadenopathy

PRIMARY HERPES OF THE PENIS

Patient Profile Uncircumcised males are especially vulnerable to severe involvement, with erosions, edema, and pain.
Age Sexually active young adults (25 percent in teen years)
Skin Symptoms Initial burning, red edematous plaque, then vesicles

Skin Lesions

TYPE Vesicles → erosions → ulcers (see Figure 95)
DISTRIBUTION Prepuce, coronal sulcus, glans, shaft

RECURRENT GENITAL HERPES IN MALES AND FEMALES

Less severe than primary, but more distressing
Skin Lesions
TYPE Vesicles on an erythematous base ⇆ erosions
ARRANGEMENT Herpetiform
DISTRIBUTION Shaft, prepuce, glans, vulva, perineum (see Figure 95)

Other Factors Pain (deep aching sensation) of the perineum may occur 2 to 3 days before appearance of the skin lesions.
Course and Prognosis The lesions disappear in 5 to 7 days. Recurrences of genital herpes are more common than labial HSV. Genital ulcer disease such as recurrent HSV infection increases risk for HIV infection.

TREATMENT OF SKIN LESIONS OF HERPES SIMPLEX

Tepid wet dressings, using aluminum subacetate solution
Acyclovir: *For primary infection,* 200 mg five times a day for 7 days. *For infrequent recurrences,* 200 mg five times a day for 5 days episodically. *For frequent recurrences,* 200–800 mg daily as prophylaxis
Caution As there is a high neonatal mortality, women with a history of genital HSV infection who are asymptomatic at the onset of labor should be advised that the risk of exposure to excretion of HSV is low and that even if inadvertent exposure does occur, the risk that their neonate will acquire an HSV infection is less than 8%. This risk can be weighed against the maternal and neonatal morbidity and the increased cost of childbirth associated with cesarean delivery. Viral cultures should be taken at weekly intervals in the final 2 months of pregnancy. If a woman is experiencing her first attack of genital HSV infection around the time of delivery, the risk that her neonate will acquire an HSV infection is likely to be substantially higher. In this circumstance, a cesarean delivery is probably prudent.

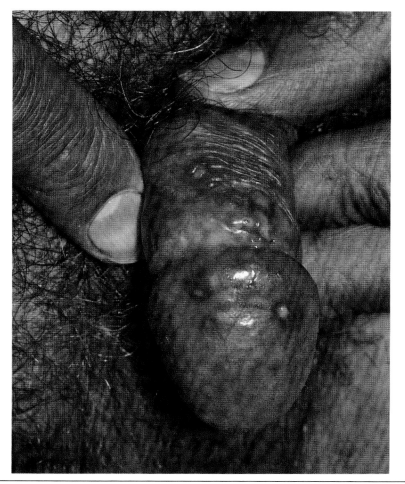

95 Herpes genitalis

Patient Profile Forty-four-year-old male salesperson

History For a year and a half, recurrent ulcers on penis

Physical Examination On inner side of preputium and on glans penis, herpetiform, grouped, shallow ulcers 2 to 3 mm in diameter. The floor of the ulcers is yellow.

Differential Diagnosis Multiple syphilitic chancres, gonococcal erosions, Candida *balanitis*, chancroid, donovanosis, lymphogranuloma inguinale

Laboratory and Special Examinations For virus: Herpesvirus hominis, type II. For spirochetes: dark-field negative. Serologic test for syphilis: negative. For bacteria: negative.

Clues Clinical aspect and laboratory examinations

Herpes Zoster

Herpes zoster is an acute localized infection caused by Varicella-zoster virus (VZV) and is characterized by unilateral pain and a vesicular or bullous eruption limited to a dermatome innervated by a corresponding sensory ganglion.

EPIDEMIOLOGY AND ETIOLOGY

Age More than 66% are over 50 years of age, while less than 10% are under 20 years

Sex and Race No differences

Incidence 300,000 annually (USA)

Other Factors Immunosuppression, especially from lymphoproliferative disorders and drugs, and local trauma to the sensory ganglia are predisposing factors for herpes zoster. Zoster is about one-third as contagious as varicella, and susceptible contacts can contract varicella. HIV-infected individuals have an 8-fold increased incidence of zoster.

HISTORY

Duration of Lesions Days to 2 to 3 weeks

Skin Symptoms Pain, tenderness, paresthesia (itching, tingling, burning) in the involved dermatome precedes the eruption by 3 to 5 days. Pain usually persists throughout the eruption, but lessens with time. Nerve involvement can occur without cutaneous zoster, i.e., zoster sine zoster.

Constitutional Symptoms Headache, malaise, fever occur in about 5% of patients

PHYSICAL EXAMINATION

Skin Lesions

TYPE
Papules (24 h)→vesicle-bulla (48 h)→ pustules (96 h)→ crusts (7 to 10 days). New lesions continue to appear for up to 1 week. Necrotic and gangrenous lesions sometimes occur.

COLOR Erythematous edematous base with superimposed clear vesicles (Figure 96), sometimes purpuric (Figure 97)

SHAPE The vesicle-bulla is oval or round

ARRANGEMENT Zosteriform (dermatomal), with herpetiform clusters of lesions (Figures 96 and 97) (see Appendix E)

DISTRIBUTION Unilateral

SITES OF PREDILECTION Thoracic (over 50%), trigeminal (10 to 20%) (Figure 98), lumbosacral and cervical (10 to 20%). In HIV-infected individuals, may be multidermatomal (contiguous or non-contiguous) and/or recurrent.

Mucous Membranes Mouth, vagina

Lymphadenopathy Regional nodes draining the area are often enlarged and tender

Sensory or Motor Nerve Changes Detectable by neurologic examination

Eye In ophthalmic zoster, nasociliary branch involvement occurs in about one-third of cases and is heralded by vesicles on the side and tip of the nose. There is usually associated conjunctivitis and occasionally keratitis scleritis or iritis. An ophthalmologist should always be consulted.

DIFFERENTIAL DIAGNOSIS

The prodromal pain of herpes zoster can mimic cardiac or pleural disease, an acute abdomen, or vertebral disease. The rash must be distinguished from zosteriform herpes simplex virus which has a different course and prognosis, especially involving the eye where herpes simplex is more pathogenic. These can be distinguished by viral culture. Contact dermatitis or localized bacterial infection should also be excluded.

PATHOPHYSIOLOGY

Varicella-zoster virus, during the course of varicella, passes from the skin lesions to the sensory nerves and travels to the sensory ganglia and establishes latent infection. It is postulated that humoral and cellular immunity to varicella-zoster virus established with primary infection persists at low levels and when this immunity ebbs, viral replication within the ganglia occurs. The virus then travels down the sensory nerve, resulting in the dermatomal pain and skin lesions. As the neuritis precedes the skin involvement, pain appears before the skin lesions are visible.

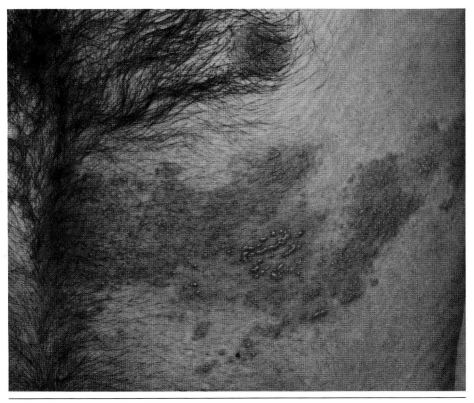

96   Herpes zoster

Patient Profile   Forty-one-year-old farmer

History   For 5 days, pain and an itching vesicular eruption of the thorax

Physical Examination   In the region of the ninth and tenth ribs the skin is patchy red and covered by closely disseminated vesicles. Except for the pain, the patient is well.

Treatment   Analgesics. The vesicles dried in 5 days; the pain disappeared gradually in 2 weeks.

COURSE AND PROGNOSIS

Postherpetic neuralgia, pain persisting after all crusts have fallen off, occurs in 10 to 15% of cases and is seen in more than one-third of patients 60 years of age or over. The highest incidence is in ophthalmic zoster. Dissemination of zoster, 20 or more lesions outside the affected or adjacent dermatomes, occurs in up to 10% of patients, usually in immunosuppressed patients. Motor paralysis is reported in up to 5% of patients, especially when *H. zoster* involves the cranial nerves.

TREATMENT

Oral corticosteroids have been shown in small controlled studies to modify the course of acute infection with a decrease in the acute neuralgia and, more importantly, a decrease in postherpetic neural-gia. This has not been shown in other controlled studies, however. Prednisone is recommended at 60 mg daily for 1 week, then tapering over 2 weeks in patients over 55 with no contraindications to steroids. Oral acyclovir in normal hosts has been shown to hasten healing and lessen acute pain if given within 48 hours of rash onset. Doses of acyclovir are 800 mg five times daily for 7 days. Decrease in postherpetic neuralgia or efficacy in ophthalmic zoster have not been shown with oral acyclovir. Current large trials with oral acyclovir and prednisone are in progress. Intravenous acyclovir or recombinant interferon alpha-2a to prevent dissemination of herpes zoster is indicated for immunosuppressed patients.

(Susan DeCoste, M.D., of Harvard Medical School helped in the preparation of this précis.)

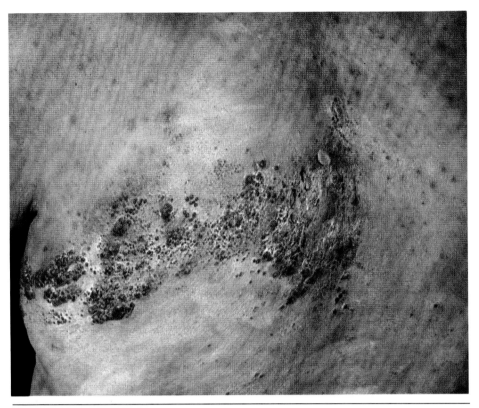

97 Herpes zoster

Patient Profile *Seventy-three-year-old male*

History *For 5 days, pain on the back and a skin eruption. The patient has chronic lymphatic leukemia.*

Physical Examination *On the left side of the back in the region of the fourth and fifth ribs, closely grouped vesicles with necrotic contents are present. Moreover, over the entire back, face, arms, and legs, widely disseminated, isolated, umbilicated vesicles with turbid content are present.*

Laboratory and Special Examinations *White blood cells: 60,000; lymphocytes: 96 percent.*

Course *Superficial necrosis developed in the region of the zoster. The skin was clear in 6 weeks; the postherpetic neuralgia lasted 2 months longer.*

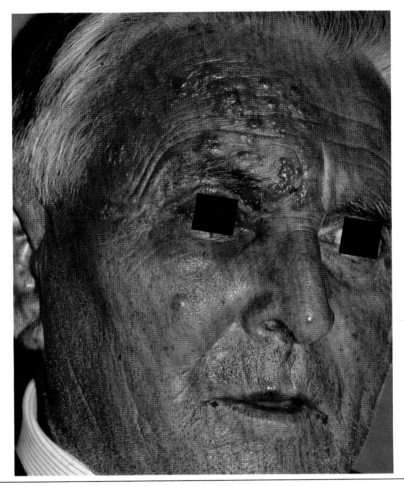

98 Herpes zoster

Patient Profile Sixty-seven-year-old male

History Five days ago headache, 2 days ago swelling of the right part of the forehead and right eye

Physical Examination In a sharply demarcated region of the right forehead and around the right eye (innervation of the first trigeminal branch), the skin is violaceous and studded with vesicles with intact roof, in part confluent. Despite involvement of the tip of the nose in this patient, there was no eye involvement. The right eyelids are edematous.

Differential Diagnosis Erysipelas

Laboratory and Special Examinations Ophthalmologic examination: no abnormalities.

XV
Syphilis

Primary Syphilis

Syphilis is a chronic, infectious disease caused by *Treponema pallidum*. It is virtually always a sexually transmitted disease. The early stages of the disease are systemic from the outset and manifested by mucocutaneous lesions that tend to ulcerate. In primary syphilis a chancre develops at the site of the inoculation and is usually accompanied by a painless regional adenopathy.

EPIDEMIOLOGY

Age In decreasing order: 20 to 39 years, 15 to 19 years, 40 to 49 years
Sex Males outnumber females 2 : 1 to 4 : 1
Other Factors In the United States 46 percent of all males with syphilis are homosexual. Syphilis is on the increase because of the availability of contraception and medical abortions and increasing promiscuity due to changing sexual behavior.

HISTORY

Contact of moist surfaces is necessary for infection.
Duration of Lesions Incubation period of 3 to 4 weeks (varies from 2 weeks to 2 months)

PHYSICAL EXAMINATION

Skin Lesions

TYPE   Chancre: buttonlike papule which develops into a *painless* ulcer with raised border, and scanty serous exudate.
COLOR   Red, "meaty-colored"
PALPATION   Firm, with *indurated* border (see Figure 99), but may not be indurated (Atypical primary syphilis: *painful* chancres, multiple ulcers or erosions, erosive balanitis, multiple lesions with thrombophlebitis of the dorsal vein)
SHAPE   Round or oval
ARRANGEMENT   Single lesion

DISTRIBUTION

Sites of predilection   Male: inner prepuce, coronal sulcus of the glans, shaft, base.

Female: cervix, vagina, vulva, clitoris, breast
Extragenital chancres   Anus or rectum, mouth, lips, tongue, fingers, toes, breasts
Miscellaneous   Physical   Findings Regional lymphadenopathy appears within 1 week. Nodes are discrete, firm, rubbery, nontender, and at first unilateral.

LABORATORY AND SPECIAL EXAMINATIONS

Dark-field Examination For spirochetes obtain tissue fluid (without red blood cells) from chancre or do a needle aspiration of enlarged regional lymph nodes.
Serologic Tests Positive reactions develop in the fourth or fifth week after infection, or 1 week after appearance of the chancre. Untreated primary syphilis has a positive FTA-ABS (fluorescent treponemal antibody absorption) test (91 percent) at 6 weeks after infection, compared to venereal disease reaction level (VDRL) (88 percent). Serologic tests become nonreactive in 1 year. (See p 263.)

TREATMENT

Benzathine penicillin G—2.4 million units total by intramuscular injection at a single session.

Patients Who Are Allergic to Penicillin

1. Tetracycline hydrochloride—500 mg 4 times a day by mouth for 15 days, *or*

2. Erythromycin (stearate, ethylsuccinate or base)—500 mg 4 times a day by mouth for 15 days

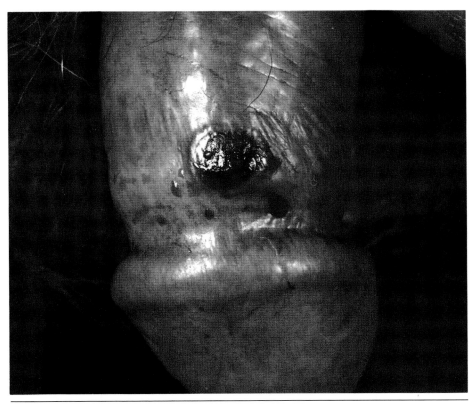

99 Primary syphilis

Patient Profile *Twenty-one-year-old male*

History *For 2 weeks, erosive lesion on penis. Not painful. General condition good. Sexual intercourse 3 weeks prior to onset of the lesion.*

Physical Examination *On the dorsum of the penile shaft near the corona is a circular, sharply outlined erosion with a small elevated border. The erosion is indurated on palpation. The inguinal lymph nodes are enlarged on both sides.*

Differential Diagnosis *Chancroid, herpes progenitalis, nonspecific penile ulcer*

Laboratory and Special Examinations *Dark-field examination:* Treponema pallidum. *Serologic tests for syphilis: initially only VDRL and FTA-ABS positive. Later, Kolmer's test, RPR, and TPI also positive.*

Clues *Indurated, painless, indolent erosion on penis, dark-field examination, serology*

Treatment *Because of known allergy to penicillin, patient was treated with oral tetracycline, 2 g daily for 14 days. Skin lesion cleared in 3 weeks; tests for syphilis became negative in 3 months. Regular supervision for 4 years revealed no abnormalities. CSF negative.*

The lesions of secondary syphilis appear 6 to 12 weeks after the onset of the chancre. In addition to a localized or generalized rash there is almost always lymph node involvement. Nontreponemal serologic tests are usually positive in high titer.

HISTORY

Syndrome appears 2 to 6 months after infection, and 6 to 8 weeks after appearance of the primary chancre.

"Acute illness" syndrome: headache, chills, feverishness, arthralgia, myalgia, malaise, photophobia.

PHYSICAL EXAMINATION

Skin Lesions

TYPE   Macules and papules 0.5 to 1.0 cm (newer lesions), round or oval (Figures 100 and 101)

COLOR   Papules: brownish red, pink (Figure 101)

PALPATION   Firm papules

SHAPE   Annular, polycyclic

ARRANGEMENT   Scattered discrete lesions (Figure 100)

DISTRIBUTION   Generalized eruption: The most common scaling papular eruption localizes especially on the head, neck, *palms,* and *soles* (Figure 100).

Associated Findings   (1) Diffuse pharyngitis or mucous patches in mouth or genitalia (small, asymptomatic, round or oval, slightly elevated, flat-topped macules and papules 0.5 to 1.0 cm in diameter, covered by thin gray membrane); or (2) acute bilateral iritis; or (3) periostitis of long bones and arthralgia or hydrarthrosis of knees or ankles without x-ray changes; or (4) meningovascular reaction; or, rarely, (5) hepatosplenomegaly, cardiac arrhythmia, nephritis, cystitis, prostatitis, gastritis

Miscellaneous   Physical   Findings   Generalized lymphadenopathy (cervical, suboccipital, inguinal, epitrochlear, axillary) and splenomegaly

DIFFERENTIAL DIAGNOSIS

Drug eruption, pityriasis rosea, viral exanthem, acute guttate psoriasis, tinea corporis

LABORATORY AND SPECIAL EXAMINATIONS

Nontreponemal serologic tests (e.g., VDRL) are always positive (>1.32). FTA-ABS is 99.2 percent positive. Beware of false-negative STS resulting from *prozone phenomenon* (undiluted serum with very high titers give negative reactions). Serologic tests become nonreactive in 24 months. STS may be negative in HIV-infected individuals. (See p 263)

TREATMENT

Same as for primary syphilis

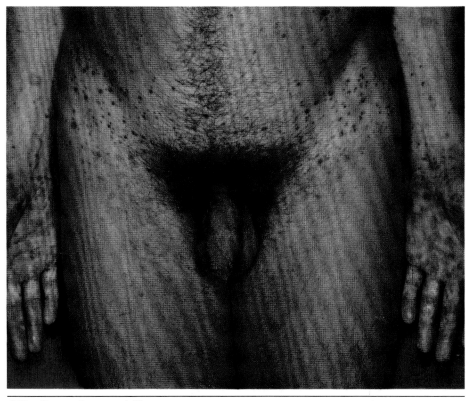

---

100 Secondary syphilis

Patient Profile Twenty-five-year-old male

History For 4 weeks, generalized nonpruritic rash, starting on the palms of the hands, subsequently spreading over arms, trunk, and soles. Slight diffuse hair loss. Otherwise no complaints. Prior to onset of the rash he had a slight, rapidly healing erosion on the penis following genitorectal intercourse.

Physical Examination On the palms of both hands, many erythematous macules, sharply outlined, varying in size from 3 to 10 mm, and on soles of feet are similar but smaller lesions, occasionally more brownish or pink-colored. There are no erosions in the mouth, on the penis, or near the anus. Lymph nodes are not enlarged. Hair loss is not pronounced and not patchy. Temperature: 38°C. General physical examination: no abnormalities

Differential Diagnosis Drug eruption, atypical pityriasis rosea, erythema multiforme

Laboratory and Special Examinations Serologic tests for syphilis: Kolmer's: + (1 : 256); VDRL: +; RPR: + (1 : 64); TPI: + ; FTA-ABS: +

Clues Eruption, especially on palms and soles, histology, serologic tests

Treatment Benzathine penicillin (2.4 million units) by intramuscular injection. Seronegativity in 3 months. One year later all tests were still negative. Two contacts were located and treated.

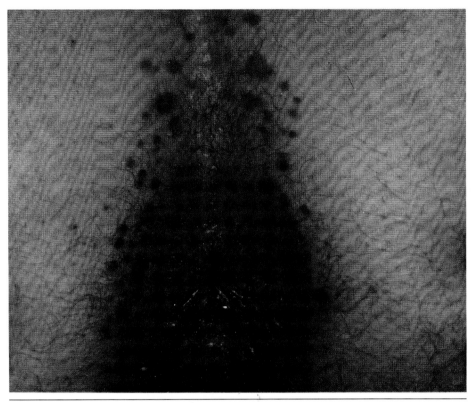

101 Primary and secondary syphilis

Patient Profile *Twenty-two-year-old homosexual male*

History *For 4 weeks, perianal rash and occasionally pain near anus*

Physical Examination *Flat, elevated, red, moist papules, partly confluent, localized around and above the anus. In the folds of the anal skin, a few fissures. Disseminated over the trunk, extremities, palms, and soles are delicate, barely visible, erythematous macules. General physical examination: no abnormalities.*

Differential Diagnosis *Eczema, candidiasis, tinea*

Laboratory and Special Examinations *Dark-field examination of moist papules and fissures: Treponema pallidum. Serologic tests for syphilis: Kolmer's, VDRL, RPR, TPI, and FTA-ABS all positive.*

Clues *Moist papules near anus, generalized exanthema, serology*

Treatment *Cleared with 2.4 million units of benzathine penicillin by intramuscular injection. VDRL was still weakly positive after 1 year; all other tests became negative. Cerebrospinal fluid examination for syphilis at that time revealed no abnormalities.*

Late syphilis is manifested in the skin, cardiovascular system, and central nervous system. In the skin, late syphilis develops in 2 to 60 years and appears as plaques or noduloulcerative lesions and gumma.

EPIDEMIOLOGY

Incidence In untreated syphilis 15 percent of patients develop late benign syphilis, mostly skin lesions, but tertiary syphilis is now very rare.

Terminology The term *gumma* (Latin, "gum") describes the rubbery lump or deep granulomatous lesion found in the subcutaneous tissue, having a tendency for necrosis and ulceration. Tubercular syphilides simulate lupus vulgaris (primary tuberculosis of the skin).

HISTORY

Duration of Lesions Three to seven years (range: 2 to 60 years); gumma develop by fifteenth year

Skin Symptoms None

PHYSICAL EXAMINATION

Skin Lesions

TUBERCULAR SYPHILIDES

Type Plaques and nodules with scars healed in the center with or without psoriasiform scales and with or without ulceration

Palpation Firm and superficial

Arrangement Serpiginous (snakelike), annular, polycyclic, scalloped borders

Distribution Solitary isolated lesions: arms (extensor aspects), back, or face

GUMMA

Type Nodule, with ulceration (Figure 102)

Palpation Soft

Arrangement Isolated

Distribution Anywhere, but especially on the scalp, face, chest, and calf

Other Physical Findings Twenty-five percent of patients have neurosyphilis or cardiovascular syphilis.

LABORATORY EXAMINATION

The serologic test for syphilis is usually highly reactive, but false-negative nontreponemal tests are possible.

COURSE

Gumma never heal spontaneously. Tubercular syphilides undergo spontaneous partial healing but new lesions appear at the periphery.

Treatment of Syphilis of More Than 1 Year's Duration (Latent Syphilis of Indeterminate or More Than 1 Year's Duration, Cardiovascular, Late Benign)

1. Benzathine penicillin G—7.2 million units total: 2.4 million units by intramuscular injection weekly for 3 successive weeks, *or*
2. Aqueous procaine penicillin G—9.0 million units total; 600,000 units by intramuscular injection daily for 15 days

Patients who are allergic to penicillin
1. Tetracycline hydrochloride—500 mg 4 times a day by mouth for 30 days, *or*
2. Erythromycin (stearate, ethylsuccinate or base)—500 mg 4 times a day by mouth for 30 days

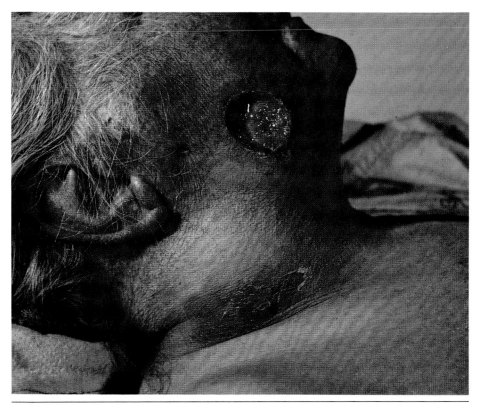

102 Tertiary (gummatous) syphilis

Patient Profile Sixty-six-year-old female

History For 8 months, gradually enlarging, red, indurated patches on the face and in the right neck. For 2 months, ulceration in one of these lesions. Otherwise no complaints.

Physical Examination In front of the right ear lobe and on the neck, two deeply indurated, red, painless nodular lesions, not sharply marginated. The lower one shows beginning central necrosis. On the right cheek is a sharply defined circular "punched out" ulcer with a necrotic base. General physical examination: no abnormalities.

Differential Diagnosis Skin tuberculosis, malignancy such as lymphoma, deep fungal infections, furuncle

Laboratory and Special Examinations Histopathology: granulomatous inflammatory reaction with large numbers of plasma cells and varying numbers of histiocytes, lymphocytes, fibroblasts, epithelioid and giant cells. Caseation necrosis. Serologic tests for syphilis: Kolmer's: +(1 : 128); VDRL: +; RPR: + (1 : 32); TPI: +. Cerebrospinal fluid examination: negative for syphilis.

Clues "Punched-out" ulcer, histology (abundant plasma cells), and serology

Treatment Procaine penicillin G in oil with 2% aluminum monostearate (PAM) 600,000 units daily on 14 subsequent days (8.4 million units total) by intramuscular injection. The skin lesions healed within a couple of months, leaving slight to moderate residual scars. Serology was greatly improved, but a few tests remained slightly positive.

False-Positive Serologic Tests for Syphilis

1. FTA-ABS can give false-positive reactions for the following reasons
   Technical error
   Inefficient sorbents
   Healthy individuals without syphilis
   Genital herpes simplex
   Pregnancy
   Lupus erythematosus (systemic or discoid)
   Alcoholic cirrhosis
   Scleroderma
   Mixed connective tissue disease

2. An even greater degree of false-positive nontreponemal reactions occur.

Transient reactors *(less than 6 months' duration)*	*Chronic reactors* *(greater than 6 months' duration)*
Technical error (low titer)	Malaria
Smallpox vaccination	Leprosy
Mycoplasma pneumonia	Systemic lupus erythematosus
Enterovirus infections	Narcotic abuse
Infectious mononucleosis	Other connective tissue disorders
Pregnancy	Elderly population
Narcotic abuse	Hashimoto's thyroiditis
Other causes commonly listed:	Rheumatoid arthritis
Advanced tuberculosis	Reticuloendothelial malignancy
Scarlet fever	Familial false-positives
Viral pneumonia	Idiopathic
Pneumonia, atypical	
Brucellosis	
Rat-bite fever	
Relapsing fever	
Leptospirosis	
Measles	
Mumps	
Lymphogranuloma venereum	
Malaria	
Trypanosomiasis	
Varicella	

3. History is important: *if* no history of possible early lesions, *or* no evidence of congenital syphilis based on patient's history, *or* no sexual exposure except to individuals who are known to have a negative STS, *then* diagnosis of false-negative STS is probably correct.

4. In Western Europe, screening of syphilis is done with TPHA and VDRL. If positive, then Reiter and FTA-ABS are done. Other treponematoses (bejel, pinta, frambesia) cannot be excluded with present serologic tests.

XVI
Insect Bites
and Infestations

Scabies

Scabies is a skin infestation of a mite, *Sarcoptes scabiei,* which is principally spread by skin-to-skin contact and causes a generalized intractable pruritus, with frequent secondary bacterial infection.

EPIDEMIOLOGY AND ETIOLOGY

Age Children (often 5 years or under) or young adults (usually acquired by sexual contact)

Other Factors Epidemics of scabies occur in cycles every 30 years. The present epidemic began in 1971 and is now subsiding.

Transmission Scabies is associated with personal skin-to-skin contact as with sexual promiscuity, crowding, poverty, or as a nosocomial outbreak. The scabies mite can remain alive for 3 to 4 days on clothing or sheets and therefore scabies may be acquired without skin-to-skin contact.

HISTORY

Duration of Lesions Primary (first) infection has an incubation period of 1 month; reinfection is followed by a hypersensitization within 24 hr.

Skin Symptoms Intense generalized intractable pruritus, a sine qua non. Intense nocturnal pruritus may occur with minimal skin lesions.

PHYSICAL EXAMINATION

Skin Lesions

TYPE

"Burrows," gray or skin-colored ridges, 0.5 to 1.0 cm in length (see Figure 103), either linear or wavy with a minute vesicle or papule at the end of the burrow

Vesicles—independent of burrows (see Figure 104)

Nodules—brownish-red, 1 to 2 cm, indurated, indolent (months)

Secondary Small urticarial papules, eczematous plaques, excoriations,

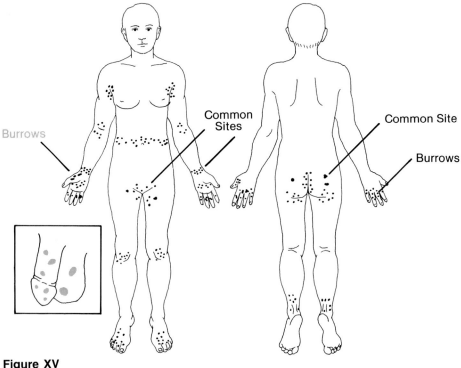

Figure XV
Scabies

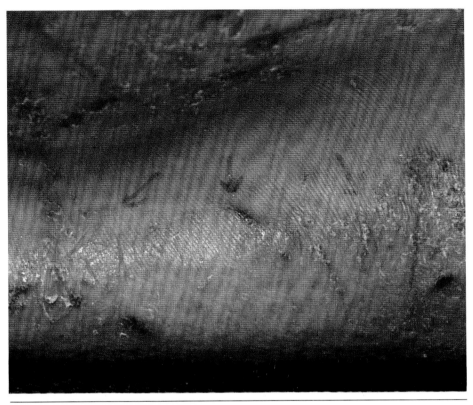

103 Scabies

Patient Profile *Twenty-year-old male*

History *For 10 weeks, gradually developed intensely pruritic eruption on the trunk, arms, hands, legs, and penis. Pruritus is worse at night. One brother has similar complaints.*

Physical Examination *On the sides of the hand and on the palm, delicate scaling areas and several slightly scaling threadlike burrows, partly erythematous. On the trunk, particularly on the buttocks, a disseminated papular eruption. On the penis (see Figure 104), some inflammatory papules covered with crusts.*

Differential Diagnosis *Dermatitis herpetiformis, nonspecified eczema, prurigo*

Laboratory and Special Examinations *Microscopic examination of roof and content of burrow (potassium hydroxide preparation):* Sarcoptes scabiei *var.* hominis, *eggs, and feces (see Figure 105).*

Clues *Pruritus (worse at night), burrows on sites of predilection, demonstration of mites and/or eggs*

Treatment *Antiscabetic cream for 12 hr, except for head. Fresh clothes and bedding. Same regimen for members of family. Afterwards: 1% hydrocortisone. Pruritus diminished rapidly, complete clearing in 3 weeks.*

and crusts of superimposed bacterial infection

(See Figure XV)

Primary lesions

Burrows—hands (palms) (90 percent) (Figure 103), wrists (flexor), penis, nipples, axillae, natal cleft
Vesicles—sides of fingers
Nodules—scrotum, penis, buttocks, groin, axillary folds, upper back

Secondary lesions Abdomen, buttocks, thighs

DIFFERENTIAL DIAGNOSIS

Assiduous search for burrows should be made in every patient with severe generalized pruritus, especially in young adults or children. Sometimes when the mite cannot be demonstrated, a "therapeutic test" will clinch the diagnosis.

SPECIAL EXAMINATION TO DETECT MITE

Look with lens for typical burrows on the finger webs, flexor aspects of wrists, and penis.
Look for "dark point" at the end of the burrow—this is the mite.

Open slowly this part of the burrow and mite will stick to the needle and will be easily transferred to the slide (see Figure 105).
If there is a nodule, biopsy will reveal portions of the mite in the corneal layer.

TREATMENT

Specific instructions must be given by the physician—and followed by the patient:

1. Bath or shower.

2. Apply to the *entire* skin (neck down) either 1% gamma-benzene hexachloride or crotamiton (especially in infants).

3. Repeat 1 and 2 *after* 24 hr *and* after 1 week.

4. Change underwear and bed sheets.

5. Take systemic antipruritics (hydroxyzine hydrochloride).

6. Itching that persists as long as 1 week later is probably related to hypersensitivity to remaining dead mites and mite products. Nevertheless, a second treatment 7 days after the first is recommended by some physicians.

7. Treat close family and personal contacts.

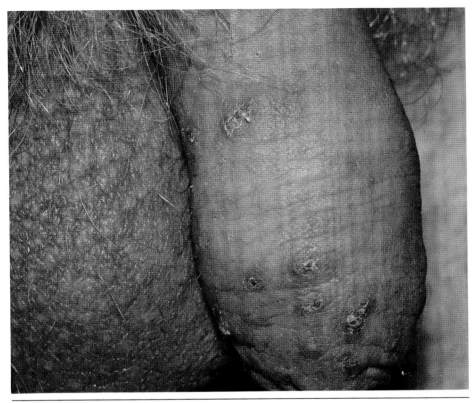

104 Scabies

Large, pruritic, crusted papules and nodules on the penis

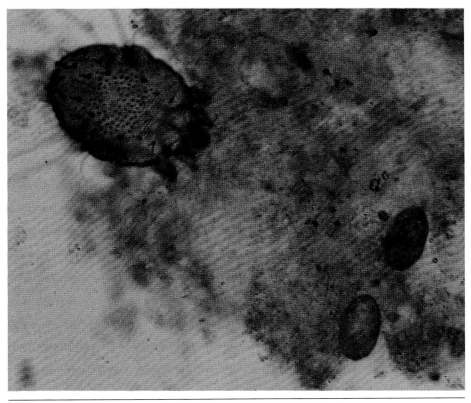

105 Scabies

Potassium hydroxide preparation of material from burrow: mite (1.3 × 0.4 mm) and eggs

Papular urticaria is an intensely pruritic eruption in which the grouped urticarial papules and papulovesicles persist for days; it occurs in young children exposed to insects, principally fleas.

EPIDEMIOLOGY AND ETIOLOGY

Age Older infants, children (under 10 years)
Season Summer in temperate climates
Etiology Dog, cat, and human fleas; mites (on dogs and cats); bedbugs; mosquitoes biting persons with hypersensitivity to insect antigens

HISTORY

Duration of Lesions Days, weeks
Skin Symptoms Intermittent mild to severe pruritus

PHYSICAL EXAMINATION

Skin Lesions

TYPE Persistent urticarial papules, often surmounted by a vesicle, usually less than 1.0 cm (lesions persist more than 48 hr). Excoriated papules.
COLOR Red
SHAPE Round
ARRANGEMENT Usually in groups of three ("breakfast, lunch, and dinner," see Figure 106)

DISTRIBUTION

Extent Generalized groups or clusters
Pattern Thighs, forearms and arms, lower part of trunk, sparing anogenital area and axillae

DIFFERENTIAL DIAGNOSIS

The diagnosis of papular urticaria, vis-à-vis chronic urticaria, is quite readily made because of the characteristically grouped, *persistent papulovesicular* lesions.

TREATMENT AND PREVENTION

Avoidance of contact with cats and dogs
Treatment of cats and dogs for fleas
Spraying the household with insecticides (e.g., malathion 1 to 4% dust) with special attention to baseboards, rugs, floors, upholstered furniture, bedframes, mattresses, and cellar

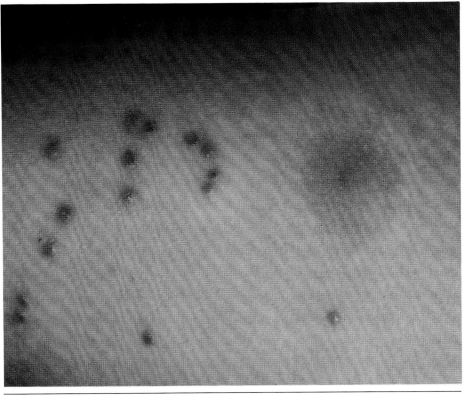

106 Papular urticaria

Patient Profile Four-year-old boy

History For 2 months, an itching eruption that impairs the sleep of the patient (and his parents)

Physical Examination Discrete papules, 1 to 3 mm in diameter, irregularly disseminated over the trunk and arms; some have a vesicle on the top, others an erosion or crust. No systemic symptoms.

Differential Diagnosis Varicella

Laboratory and Special Examinations Mite was found in the hair of a pet dog.

Clue Typical grouping of lesions

Treatment Antipruritic lotion containing menthol. Treatment of the dog with an insect spray. The eruption cleared in 3 weeks.

Bullous Insect Bite

A bullous insect bite is a relatively common reaction occurring on the lower legs in persons (usually children) who are hypersensitive to mosquitoes or horseflies. Repeated episodes occur in the same person in subsequent summers.

TREATMENT

Leave the roof of the bulla in place; empty the bulla and apply antibacterial ointment.

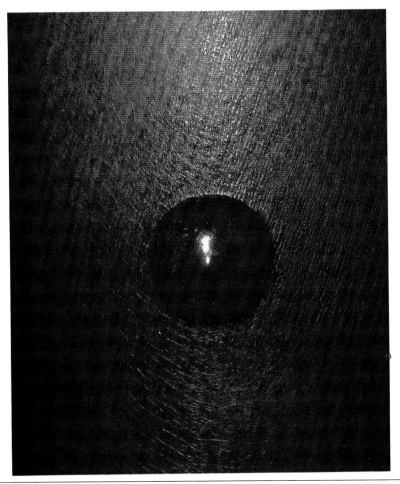

107 Bullous eruption caused by an insect bite

Patient Profile Fifty-six-year-old Indonesian female homemaker

History Patient migrated 3 years ago to the Netherlands. Since then, intermittently on different parts of body, itching papules that develop within a few days into blisters. Patient noticed that sometimes the eruption is preceded by an insect bite.

Physical Examination On the right lower leg, a tense bulla, 2.5 cm in diameter, filled with a clear yellow liquid. On the right thigh and arm, papules with a vesicle on top.

Differential Diagnosis Dermatitis herpetiformis, drug eruption

Laboratory and Special Examinations Smear of blister content: a few leukocytes, an occasional eosinophil. Histopathology of arm: nonspecific perivascular inflammation immunofluorescence negative.

Clues History, absence of symptoms of an autoimmune bullous disease

Pathophysiology Hyperergic reaction to insects, probably Culex species.

Treatment Antipruritic lotion topically, antihistamines orally, and an insect repellent. Patient gradually became symptom-free.

XVII

Benign Neoplasms

Epidermis
Melanocytes
Blood Vessels

This very common, hereditary, benign tumor is usually pigmented; it occurs after age 30, especially on the trunk and face.

EPIDEMIOLOGY AND ETIOLOGY

Age Rarely before 30 years of age
Sex Slightly more common and more profuse in males
Other Features Autosomal dominant trait

HISTORY

Duration of Lesions Usually months to years
Skin Symptoms Rarely pruritic; tender if secondarily infected

PHYSICAL EXAMINATION

Skin Lesions

TYPE

Early Small, 1- to 3-mm, barely elevated papule or plaque with or without pigment. The surface shows, with 7X to 10X magnification, fine stippling like a thimble.
Later Plaque with warty surface and "stuck on" appearance (see Figures 108 and 109); with a hand lens (7X to 10X) horn cysts can invariably be seen on the surface. Size from 1.0 to 6.0 cm (see Figure 110)
SHAPE Round, oval
ARRANGEMENT Scattered, discrete lesions

DISTRIBUTION Isolated lesion or generalized
SITES OF PREDILECTION Face, trunk, upper extremities

DIFFERENTIAL DIAGNOSIS

Early "flat" lesions confused with *solar lentigo* or *spreading pigmented actinic keratosis* (surface of seborrheic keratosis is more verrucous, also horn cysts are present); larger pigmented lesions are easily mistaken for *pigmented basal cell carcinoma* or *malignant melanoma* (only biopsy will settle this)

DERMATOPATHOLOGY

Site Epidermis
Process Proliferation of immature keratinocytes (with marked papillomatosis) and melanocytes, formation of horn cysts

TREATMENT

Light electrocautery will permit the whole lesion to appear to be easily rubbed off. Then the base can be lightly cauterized to prevent recurrence. Cryotherapy is effective, but recurrences are more frequent than when electrocautery is used.

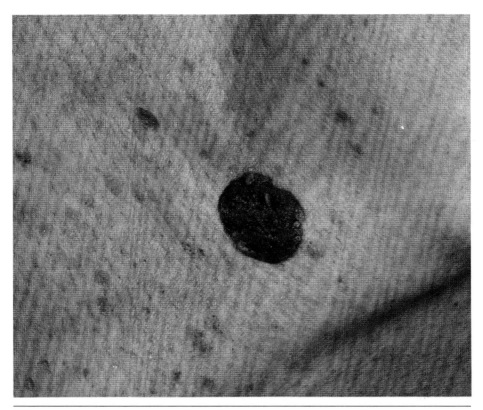

108 Seborrheic keratosis

Patient Profile Seventy-six-year-old retired carpenter

History For many years, an itching brown tumor on the right shoulder

Physical Examination A slightly elevated, somewhat warty, keratotic brown tumor, sharply outlined, no variegation in color, 2 cm in diameter. It seems as if the lesion is superficially "stuck on" the skin.

Differential Diagnosis Melanocytic nevus, melanoma

Laboratory and Special Examinations Histology: benign basal cell papilloma with hyperkeratosis and pigmentation.

Clues Waxy (greasy) keratotic surface, "stuck on" appearance, histology

Treatment Curettage and cryotherapy

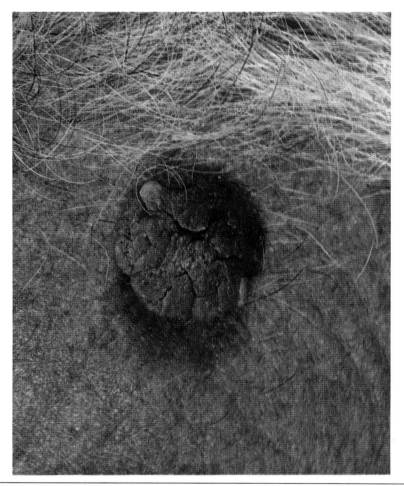

109 Seborrheic keratosis

Patient Profile Sixty-year-old farmer

History For 8 years, a nonprogressive warty tumor on the right temple. Two weeks ago an erythematous halo developed around the tumor, accompanied by tenderness and itching.

Physical Examination The tumor is slightly elevated, 2.5 cm in diameter, and has a warty, waxy keratotic surface. The tumor seems to be "stuck on" the skin (compare with Figure 108). The color is grayish-brown without variegation. The lesion is partly surrounded by a narrow erythematous zone.

Differential Diagnosis Lentigo maligna, nodular melanoma

Laboratory and Special Examinations Histology: benign basal cell papilloma with inflammatory reaction in the dermis, compatible with an irritated seborrheic keratosis.

Clues "Stuck-on" appearance, greasy keratosis, no variegation in pigmentation

Treatment Light electrocautery and curettage under local anesthesia

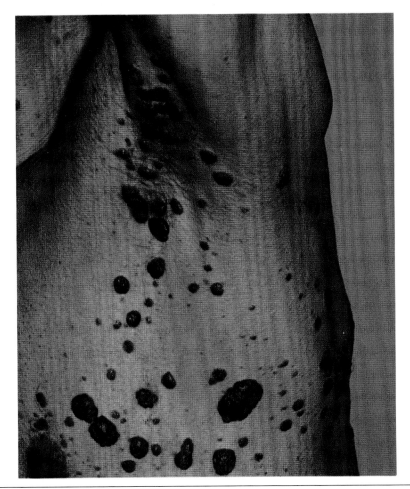

110 Multiple seborrheic keratoses

Patient Profile Seventy-six-year-old male

History For 15 years, steadily increasing number of warty lesions on trunk, occasionally pruritic

Physical Examination A large number of pigmented lesions, disseminated over the chest and back. Most lesions are dark brown, waxy keratotic, sharply demarcated, often somewhat papillomatous, varying in size from 0.5 to 3 cm. Some are light brown or yellowish and flatter. All have a "stuck-on" appearance, giving the impression that they can be "picked off" the skin.

Differential Diagnosis Melanoma, melanocytic nevi

Laboratory and Special Examinations A biopsy is not required in this typical case.

Clues "Stuck-on" warty appearance, no variegation in color

Treatment On patient's request, a large number of the lesions were treated with liquid nitrogen, resulting in a temporary clearing. Recurrences within 6 to 12 months

Keratoacanthoma

Keratoacanthoma is a self-healing, rapidly developing, benign epithelial neoplasm that simulates squamous cell carcinoma.

EPIDEMIOLOGY

Age Over 50 years; rare below 20 years
Sex Males
Race Caucasians, rare in Asians

HISTORY

Duration of Lesions Rapid growth, achieving a size of 2.5 cm within 6 weeks
Skin Symptoms None

PHYSICAL EXAMINATION

Skin Lesions

TYPE Nodule, dome-shaped often with a central keratotic plug (Figure 111)
COLOR Skin-colored or slightly red
PALPATION Firm but not hard
SIZE AND SHAPE 2.5 cm (1.0 to 10.0 cm) or round
DISTRIBUTION Isolated single lesion
SITES OF PREDILECTION Cheeks, nose, ears, and hands (dorsa)

DIFFERENTIAL DIAGNOSIS

Squamous cell carcinoma—a wedge biopsy must be done as it is impossible to make a clinical distinction between keratoacanthoma and squamous cell carcinoma

DERMATOPATHOLOGY

Site Epidermis
Process Proliferative. Central, large, irregularly shaped crater filled with keratin. The surrounding epidermis extends in a liplike manner over the sides of the crater. The keratinocytes are atypical with many mitoses, and many are dyskeratotic.

PATHOPHYSIOLOGY

This neoplasm is probably caused by a virus, but there is no proof. Other etiologic factors include ultraviolet radiation and chemical carcinogens (industrial: pitch and tar).

COURSE AND PROGNOSIS

Spontaneous regression in 2 to 6 months or sometimes over 1 year

TREATMENT

The regressed lesion may result in a rather disfiguring scar so that surgical excision or curettage followed by electrocautery is recommended. Histologic confirmation of the clinical diagnosis is important as this lesion can mimic a squamous cell carcinoma.

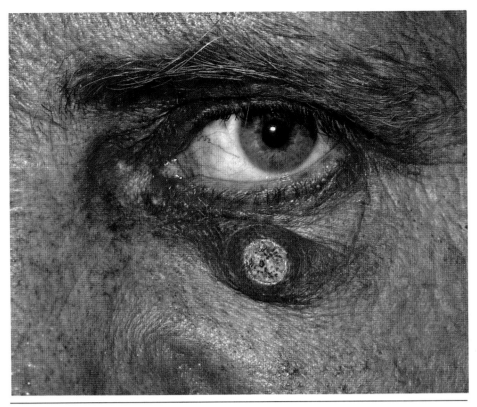

111 Keratoacanthoma

Patient Profile Forty-eight-year-old male

History For 12 days, an asymptomatic tumor under the left eye

Physical Examination Oval, erythematous violaceous tumor under left eye, 3 cm in diameter, with a horny plug in center

Differential Diagnosis Squamous cell carcinoma

Dermatopathology Histopathology: the acanthotic squamous cell layer shows a liplike turnback where it folds over a horny plug. The epithelium delimiting the horny plug is markedly acanthotic and protrudes with buds and finer strands into surrounding tissue. No atypical keratinocytes nor individual cell keratinization. The tumor mass is surrounded by a dense round cell infiltration. Pathologic diagnosis: probably keratoacanthoma, but squamous cell carcinoma cannot be excluded.

Clues Histopathology, rapid growth

Course Cleared without any treatment in 5 weeks.

Solar Lentigo

Solar lentigo is a circumscribed 1.0- to 3.0-cm brown macule resulting from a localized proliferation of melanocytes as a result of chronic exposure to sunlight.

EPIDEMIOLOGY AND ETIOLOGY

Age   Usually over 40 years, but may occur at 30 years in sunny climates

Sex   No data available, probably equal incidence

Race   Most common in Caucasians, but seen also in Asians

Predisposing Factors   Generally correlated with Skin Phototypes I to III and duration and intensity of solar exposure (see Appendix D)

PHYSICAL EXAMINATION

Skin Lesions

TYPE   Strictly macular, 1 to 3 cm, as large as 5.0 cm

COLOR   Light yellow, light brown, or dark brown; variegated mix of brown and not uniform color as in café-au-lait spots. When dark brown areas develop (rare), it is called *lentigo maligna,* a premalignant lesion.

SHAPE   Round, oval, with slightly irregular border

ARRANGEMENT   Often scattered, discrete lesions

DISTRIBUTION   Pattern—exclusively exposed areas: forehead, cheeks, nose, dorsa of hands and forearms, upper back, and chest

DERMATOPATHOLOGY

Site   Epidermis

Process   Proliferative. Club-shaped elongated rete ridges which show hypermelanosis and increased number of melanocytes in the basal layer

DIFFERENTIAL DIAGNOSIS AND TREATMENT

"Flat," acquired, brown lesions of the exposed skin of the face, which may on cursory examination appear to be similar, have distinctive features:

Solar lentigo, the most frequently observed lesion, has a medium brown color and is completely flat and without evidence of epidermal change, even when carefully examined with a hand lens and oblique lighting. The lesions may gradually enlarge to 3 to 4 cm or more and completely disappear for 1 to 3 years following very short exposures (10 s) to liquid nitrogen applied with a cotton tip.

Seborrheic keratosis may be indistinguishable in its early stages from solar lentigo, but usually epidermal change is barely perceptible in seborrheic keratoses when examined with a hand lens and oblique lighting. (See Figures 108–110.)

Lentigo maligna is completely flat, without any epidermal alteration, and simulates solar lentigo except for a distinct variegation of color: brown, dark brown, and flecks of black. These lesions should always be biopsied and, if proved histologically, excised with a narrow margin; usually a split-thickness graft is necessary.

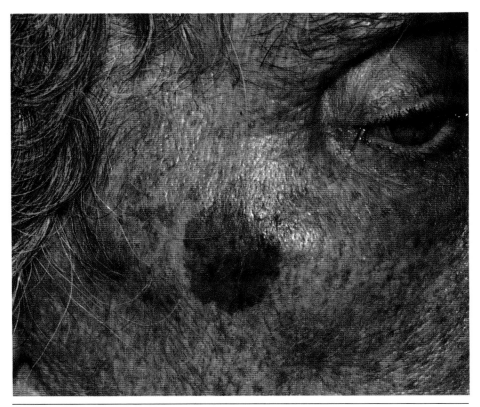

112   Solar lentigo

Patient Profile   Seventy-one-year-old farmer's wife

History   For many years, a gradually developing brown spot on right cheek

Physical Examination   In the right zygomatous region, a round, sharply demarcated macule varying from light to dark brown. The surrounding skin shows patchy hyperpigmentation and telangiectases, as found after lifelong sun exposure.

Differential Diagnosis   Lentigo maligna, seborrheic keratosis. The absence of black spots in the macule excludes a lentigo maligna, the absence of elevation a seborrheic keratosis. The clinical clues were sufficient to obviate the necessity of a biopsy.

Treatment   The elderly woman was not interested in a treatment for cosmetic reasons. Patients who are eager for cosmetic improvement may be treated with 5-fluorouracil cream or liquid nitrogen.

Common Melanocytic Nevocellular Nevi (Moles)

Melanocytic nevocellular nevi are small (less than 1.5 cm), circumscribed, acquired pigmented macules or papules comprised of groups of melanocytes or melanocytic nevus cells located in the epidermis, dermis, and rarely subcutaneous tissue.

EPIDEMIOLOGY

Race

One of the most common acquired new growths in Caucasians (over two-thirds have one or more), less common in blacks or pigmented peoples, and infrequent in fair-skinned persons (Skin Type I) (see Appendix D).

Dysplastic nevi, which are precursor lesions of malignant melanoma, occur in 30 percent of patients with primary melanoma and in 6 percent of their family members.

HISTORY

Duration of Lesions These lesions, which are commonly called *moles,* appear in early childhood and reach a maximum in young adulthood. There is a gradual involution of lesions and most disappear by age 60 (the dermal melanocytic nevocellular nevus does not disappear).

Skin Symptoms Nevocellular nevi are asymptomatic, and if a lesion begins to itch or is tender, it should be carefully followed, as pruritus, for example, may be an early indication of malignant change.

CLASSIFICATION

Nevocellular nevi (NCN) can be classified according to the site of the clusters of nevus cells.

Junctional Malanocytic NCN Cells at dermal—epidermal junction above basement membrane (see Figure 113)

Dermal Melanocytic NCN Cells exclusively in the dermis (see page 294 and Figure 116)

Compound Melanocytic NCN A combination of the histologic features of junctional and dermal

Clark's Melanocytic Nevus See page 292 and Figure 115

Junctional Melanocytic Nevocellular Nevi

(Figure 113, lesions at three and six o'clock)

Skin Lesions

TYPE Macule, or only very slightly raised

SIZE If larger than 1.5 cm, the mole is congenital not acquired, or dysplastic mole

COLOR Uniform tan, brown, or dark brown

SHAPE Round or oval with smooth regular borders

ARRANGEMENT Scattered discrete lesions, usually too many to count

DISTRIBUTION Random

SITES OF PREDILECTION Palms and soles, trunk, upper extremities, face, lower extremities

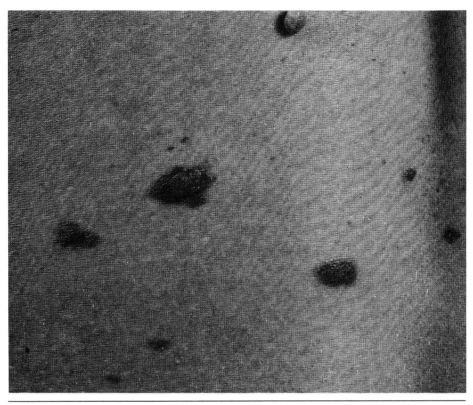

113   Multiple melanocytic nevi

Patient Profile   Eighteen-year-old male

History   For many years, a large number of asymptomatic pigmented moles on the trunk and extremities. New lesions have developed in the past 2 years.

Physical Examination   Disseminated over the chest, back, and arms are approximately 30 light brown, slightly elevated tumors, ranging in size from 3 to 7 mm. Some are papillomatous, others flat. The margins are sharp, occasionally irregular. Patient has Skin Phototype II.

Laboratory and Special Examinations   Biopsies: flat, dark-colored lesion—junctional nevus; elevated, pale-brown lesion—compound nevus

Compound Melanocytic Nevocellular Nevi (Figure 114)

Skin Lesions Same color and shape as junctional melanocytic NCN except that they are not commonly seen on the palms and soles and are always distinctively elevated

TREATMENT

Indications for removal of acquired melanocytic NCN are

1. *Site*—lesions on the scalp, soles, all mucous membranes, anogenital area; any mole that is constantly exposed to trauma

2. *Color*—if color is or becomes variegated

3. *Border*—if irregularly irregular borders are present

4. *Symptoms*—if lesion begins to persistently itch, hurt, or bleed

These criteria are based on anatomic sites at risk for change of acquired nevi to malignant melanoma *or* on changes in individual lesions (color, border) that indicate the development of a focus of cells with *dysplasia,* the precursor of malignant melanoma. Clark's Melanocytic Nevi are *usually* larger than 7 mm, and darker, with distinctive variegation of color (tan, brown), and have irregularly irregular borders. These lesions occur over the trunk and upper extremities, but also on the buttocks, groin, scalp, and female breasts.

Melanocytic NCN should always be excised for histologic diagnosis and for definitive treatment. Electrocautery should never be used for removal.

See Recommendations for the Management of Pigmented Lesions to Facilitate Early Diagnosis of Malignant Melanoma in Appendix F.

The Clark Melanocytic Nevus (So-called Dysplastic Nevus) (Figure 115)

Clark melanocytic nevi (CMN) are well-circumscribed, acquired, disordered proliferations of variably atypical melanocytes that arise de novo or more frequently as part of a compound melanocytic nevus. CMN differ from common acquired nevi and are clinically distinctive and have characteristic histologic features. CMN are regarded as potential precursors of superficial spreading malignant melanoma.

EPIDEMIOLOGY AND ETIOLOGY

Prevalence CMN occur in almost every patient with familial cutaneous melanoma and in 30% to 50% of patients with sporadic (nonfamilial) melanoma and 5% of the general population.

Race White persons. Data on persons with brown or black skin are not available.

Age CMN develop by age 20 years and appear first in childhood just before puberty. New lesions continue to develop over a period of years in affected persons, in contrast to common acquired melanocytic nevi which do not usually appear after middle age.

Heredity Autosomal dominant or sporadic

DERMATOPATHOLOGY

Site Dermal-epidermal junction and dermis

Process Hyperplasia and proliferation of randomly "atypical" melanocytes in "lentiginous" and/or "epithelioid" pattern.

COURSE AND SIGNIFICANCE

Anatomic association (in contiguity) of dysplastic nevi has been observed in 36% of sporadic primary melanomas, in about 69% of familial primary melanomas, and in 94% of melanomas in patients with dysplastic nevus syndrome and familial melanoma.

The lifetime risks for developing primary malignant melanoma are estimated to be:

General population 0.7%
Familial dysplastic nevus syndrome with two blood relatives with melanoma. . . . 100%
All other patients who have dysplastic nevi syndrome. 18%

It is obvious that all patients with familial dysplastic nevus syndrome need to be carefully followed (preferably every 2 to 6 months) for changes in existing dysplastic nevi (increase in size, changes in pigmentation, etc.). Only suspicious lesions or lesions that are changing need be excised.

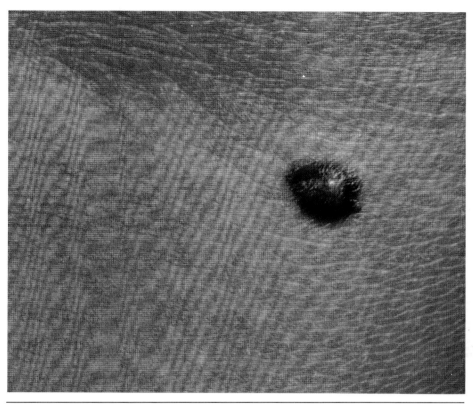

114   Compound melanocytic nevus

Patient Profile   Three-year-old boy

History   For 18 months, in bend of left knee, an asymptomatic pigmented mole that increased in size in the past months

Physical Examination   Nodular tumor of firm consistency, 50 × 35 mm, slightly elevated, dark brown to black, smooth surface without defects, surrounded by a narrow light-brown halo

Differential Diagnosis   Blue nevus, hemangioma, melanoma

Laboratory and Special Examinations   Histology: nests of melanocytes in dermis, and also in the epidermis above the basement membrane. No signs of malignancy.

Clues   The intense dark color is suggestive of junctional activity; the nodular appearance points to a dermal nevus. Absence of variegation in color argues against melanoma.

Treatment   Excision because the possibility of a melanoma could not be excluded

COMPARATIVE CLINICAL FEATURES

	Clark Melanocytic Nevus	*Common Acquired Melanocytic Nevus*
Number	One or many. Dozens or uncountable, especially in familial melanoma	One or many, average of 12–15 lesions per person. Thirty percent of white adults have no nevi
Distribution	Any location (trunk predominates) including covered areas (scalp, buttocks, female breasts)	Any location. Sun-exposed areas of trunk and extremities, rare on buttocks and female breasts
˙Type	Macules and papules, even if large (>6.0 mm), there is often only slight focal elevation (surface assessed by side-lighting)	Small lesions (junctional nevi) are macules and larger lesions (6.0 mm) are usually uniformly elevated (papules or plaques)
˙Size	Usually up to 15 mm. Lesions above 6.0 mm to be regarded as CMN or congenital nevi	Most less than 10 mm
˙Color:		
HUE	Brown (dark or medium), tan (pink)	Brown (medium or dark), tan
PATTERN	Irregular display of brown and dark brown	Uniform or orderly pattern
Shape	Round, oval, or ellipsoid	Round or oval
˙Outline of Border	Indistinct margin with the normal skin and/or irregular border	Sharply demarcated, regular border

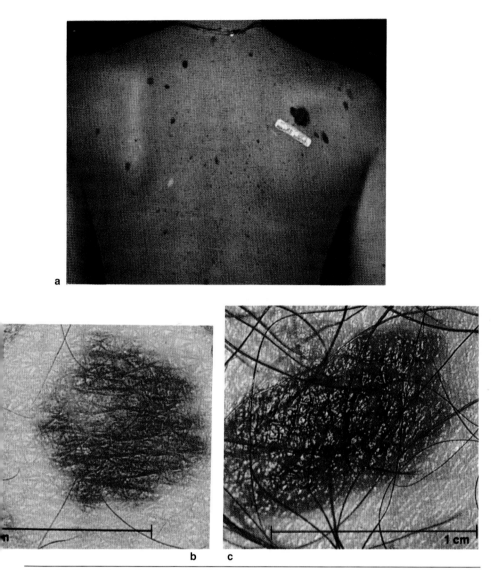

a

b   c

115 Malignant melanoma–Clark's melanocytic nevus (dysplastic nevus syndrome)

(a) This 28-year-old woman gave a history of a rapidly growing (3 to 6 months), asymptomatic lesion on her right scapular area. Her mother had melanoma and both mother and siblings had many dark "moles." Diagnosis: (1) Superficial spreading melanoma, level IV, 4.75 mm. (2) Regional nodes—of 32 removed, 1 was positive. (3) Dysplastic nevus syndrome with family history of melanoma. Primary lesion and many dark "moles" on back. (b) Round essentially macular lesions in which the slightly elevated area is present at 12:00 o'clock. The elevation is detectable only by oblique lighting. Note striking variegation of color with tan, brown, and pink areas. (c) This lesion is more obviously elevated in the central portion. Note "pebbly" surface. Both lesions have indistinct and irregular borders. (From Dermatologic Capsule & Comment 7(4):4, 1985, with permission.)

Dermal Melanocytic Nevocellular Nevi (Figure 116)

SKIN LESIONS

Type Papule (Figures 115 and 116)
Color Skin-colored, tan, brown, or flecks of brown, often with telangiectasia
Shape Round, dome-shaped (Figures 115 and 116)
Distribution More common on the face and neck, but can occur on the trunk or extremities

Other Features Usually appear in the second or third decade and do not spontaneously disappear

DIFFERENTIAL DIAGNOSIS

Dermal nevi are sometimes indistinguishable from basal cell carcinoma.

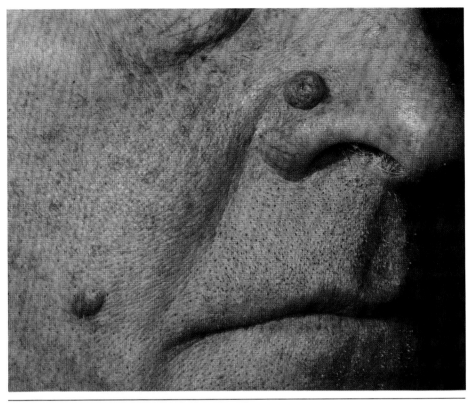

116 Dermal melanocytic nevus

Patient Profile Sixty-one-year-old carpenter

History For about 20 years, two tumors on the right cheek

Physical Examination On right ala of nose, a soft, pale-red, pea-sized tumor, with a shallow sagging in the center

Differential Diagnosis Dermal melanocytic nevus, fibroma, nodular basal cell carcinoma

Dermatopathology In the dermis nest, closely grouped, large polygonal cells with large pale nuclei: dermal melanocytic nevus.

Clues History; soft, not hard, as in basal cell carcinoma

Treatment Excision

CONGENITAL NEVOMELANOCYTIC NEVUS (CNN)

CNN are pigmented lesions of the skin usually present at birth. CNN may be any size from very small to very large, covering large portions of the body. All CNN, regardless of size, may be precursors of malignant melanoma.

EPIDEMIOLOGY

Sex Equal prevalence in males and females

Race All races

Prevalence CNN present in 1.0% of newborns—majority <3.0 cm in diameter. Larger varieties are present in 1:2,000 to 1:20,000 newborns. Lesions ≥9.9 cm have a prevalence of 1:20,000 and giant CNN (occupying a major portion of a major anatomic site) occur in 1:500,000 newborns.

PHYSICAL EXAMINATION

Small and Large CNN

TYPE Plaque with or without coarse hairs

BORDERS Sharply demarcated or merging imperceptibly with surrounding skin, regular or irregular contours

SURFACE May or may not have altered skin surface ("pebbly," mammillated, rugose, cerebriform, bulbous, tuberous, or lobular). These surface changes are more frequently observed in those lesions that extend into the reticular dermis (so-called deep CNN).

COLOR Light or dark brown

SIZE Nevomelanocytic nevi >1.5 cm in diameter should be regarded as probably CNN when history is not available.

DISTRIBUTION Isolated, discrete lesion at any site

Very Large ("Giant") CNN

NUMBER Giant CNN often present as a single, very large lesion and multiple smaller lesions.

TYPE Plaque with surface distortion, often with focal nodules, and often with coarse hair

COLOR Light or medium brown, or dark brown, often with a variegated pigment pattern.

SIZE Entire segments of the trunk, extremities, head or neck

DISTRIBUTION Present in any region of the body

Giant CNN of the head and neck may be associated with involvement of the leptomeninges.

DIFFERENTIAL DIAGNOSIS

Small CNN are virtually indistinguishable clinically from common acquired nevomelanocytic nevi except for size—lesions >1.5 cm may be presumed to be either CNN or Clark's dysplastic melanocytic nevi. Without a good history or histology (?), it may not be possible to ascertain the age of onset of a nevomelanocytic nevus <1.5 cm in diameter.

LABORATORY AND SPECIAL EXAMINATIONS

Histopathology

SMALL AND LARGE CNN Unlike the common acquired nevomelanocytic nevus, the nevomelanocytes in CNN tend to occur in the skin appendages (eccrine ducts, hair follicles, sebaceous glands), and into nerve fascicles and/or arrector pilorum muscles, blood vessels (especially veins), lymphatic vessels, and extend into the lower two-thirds of the reticular dermis and deeper.

VERY LARGE OR GIANT CNN A similar histopathology to small and large CNN but the nevomelanocytes may extend into the muscle, bone, dura mater, and cranium.

COURSE AND PROGNOSIS

Small CNN The lifetime risk of developing malignant melanoma is 1–5%.

Very Large or Giant CNN The lifetime risk for development of melanoma in large CNN has been estimated to be at least 6.3%; in 50% of patients who develop melanoma in large CNN, the diagnosis is made between ages 3 to 5 years.

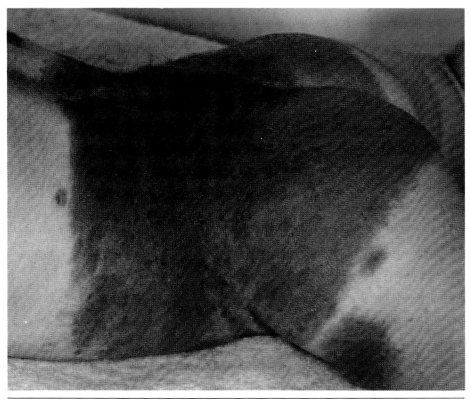

117   Congenital pigmented melanocytic nevus

Patient Profile   Two-day-old boy

History   Since birth. Family history noncontributory

Physical Examination   On the lower parts of the back, abdomen, buttocks, and thighs is an extensive, slightly indurated, brown-colored area. Scattered over the lesion are darker-colored areas. Hair growth is somewhat increased. A large number of similar but much smaller separate lesions are present on other parts of the trunk, extremities, and scalp.

MANAGEMENT

Small and Large CNN   Excision, with full-thickness skin graft, swing flaps, or tissue expanders; for some lesions, photographic follow-up for life.

Giant CNN   Ideally, excision. Individual considerations are necessary (size, location, degree of loss of function or of mutilation).

(Dr. Arthur R. Rhodes assisted in the preparation of this précis)

Halo Nevus (Sutton's Leukoderma Acquisitum Centrifugum)

EPIDEMIOLOGY AND ETIOLOGY

Age First three decades
Race and Sex All races, both sexes
Incidence In patients with vitiligo, 1 to 50 percent
Family History Halo nevi occur in siblings and with history of vitiligo in family
Associated Disorders Vitiligo, metastatic melanoma (around lesions and around nevus cell nevi)
"Halo" Depigmentation around Other Lesions Blue nevus, congenital garment nevus cell nevus, Spitz's juvenile nevus, verruca plana, primary melanoma, dermatofibroma, and neurofibroma

HISTORY

Three Stages

1. Development (in months) of halo around preexisting nevus cell nevus

2. Disappearance (months to years) of nevus cell nevus

3. Repigmentation (months to years) of halo

PHYSICAL EXAMINATION

Skin Lesions

TYPE Papular brown nevus cell nevus (5.0 mm) with halo of sharply marginated hypomelanosis (see Figure 118)
SHAPE Oval hypomelanosis (see Figure 118)

ARRANGEMENT Scattered discrete lesions (1 to 90)
DISTRIBUTION Trunk (same as distribution of nevus cell nevus)

DERMATOPATHOLOGY AND ELECTRON MICROSCOPY

Nevus Cell Nevus Dermal or compound nevus surrounded by lymphocytic infiltrate (lymphocytes and histiocytes) around and between nevus cells. Nevus cells develop evidence of cell damage and disappear.
Halo Epidermis Decrease or absence of melanin and melanocytes (as shown by electron microscopy)

PATHOPHYSIOLOGY

Immunologic phenomena are responsible for the dynamic changes through the action of circulating cytotoxic antibodies and/or cytotoxic lymphocytes. This disease awaits a reevaluation using newer techniques (immunofluorescence, status of Langerhans cells, T cells, etc.).

TREATMENT

None. The lesions undergo spontaneous resolution. The nevus cell nevi must always be evaluated for clinical criteria of malignancy (variegation of pigment and irregular borders) as a "halo" can and does occasionally develop around primary malignant melanoma.

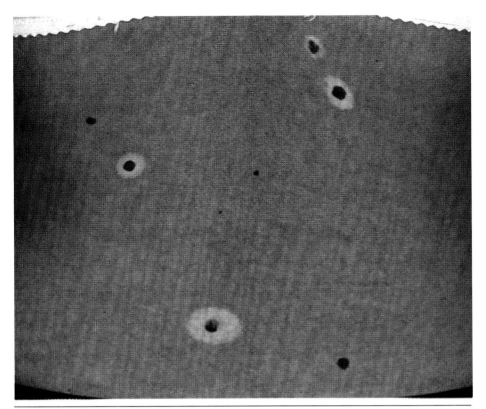

118   Halo nevi
Leukoderma acquisitum centrifugum
Sutton's nevus

Patient Profile   Fifteen-year-old girl

History   For many years, multiple lesions disseminated over the back, chest, and abdomen. For a couple of months, white areas have developed around some of the moles.

Physical Examination   Disseminated over the back are nine brown pigmented lesions, 2 to 5 mm in diameter, slightly elevated, and sharply demarcated. Four are surrounded by a sharply marginated, 2- to 5-mm white zone.

Differential Diagnosis   Melanoma with leukoderma (hypomelanosis), nevi associated with vitiligo

Laboratory and Special Examinations   Histology: benign compound melanocytic nevus.

Treatment   None. One year later two of the nevi within the hypomelanotic areas had disappeared and there was a beginning of repigmentation. The other halo nevi were unchanged.

Nevus Flammeus (Port-Wine Stain)

These nevi are irregularly shaped, red or violaceous macules that are present at birth and never disappear; the pigmentation reflects permanent dilatation of capillaries in the dermis.

EPIDEMIOLOGY

Age Congenital

HISTORY

Skin Symptoms None

PHYSICAL EXAMINATION

Skin Lesions

TYPE Macule. Papules or nodules can develop in adulthood, leading to quite marked disfigurement.
COLOR Varying hues of pink to purple (see Figure 119)
SHAPE Irregular. Large lesions follow a dermatomal distribution and rarely cross the midline.
DISTRIBUTION Localized or regional (e.g., the entire leg)
PATTERN Dermatomal
Miscellaneous Findings Tissue hypertrophy and enlargement of the leg or arm, genitalia, and lips may occur, occasionally with gross disfigurement.

DIFFERENTIAL DIAGNOSIS

Port-wine stains may be a manifestation of a larger vascular developmental defect, the *Sturge-Weber syndrome,* which includes ocular (glaucoma) and intracranial vascular ectasia (leptomeninges), and involves all or part of the trigeminal nerve unilaterally. Seizures frequently occur and mental retardation is common.

DERMATOPATHOLOGY

Site Capillaries
Process Developmental defect leading to ectasia of capillaries. No proliferation of endothelial cells

RADIOGRAPHY

Axial tomography to detect intracranial calcification, which may be associated with a rather small port-wine stain

COURSE AND PROGNOSIS

Involution of the port-wine mark does not occur; purplish protruding nodules may develop.

TREATMENT

Port-wine stains are easily covered with makeup such as Cover-Mark.
Treatment with laser is effective and increasingly available.

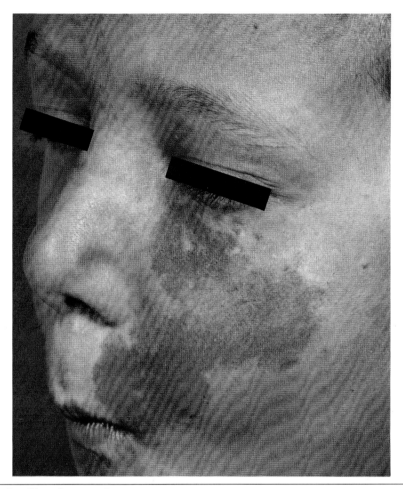

119 Capillary hemangioma
Port-wine stain
Nevus flammeus

Patient Profile Five-year-old boy

History Since birth, an extensive red discoloration of the skin on the left cheek. The condition has not changed fundamentally.

Physical Examination On the left cheek is an extensive, macular, red to purplish-red colored area, not indurated or elevated, blanching under pressure. On close examination numerous telangiectases are seen.

Laboratory and Special Examinations Ophthalmic and neurologic examinations revealed no abnormalities.

Treatment Cosmetic covering was not desired. Laser therapy was not available at that time. Three years later the condition was unchanged.

Angiomatous Nevus (Strawberry Nevus)

An angiomatous nevus is a soft, bright red, vascular nodule that develops at birth or soon after birth and disappears spontaneously by the fifth year.

HISTORY

Duration of Lesion Lesion appears within the first month of life in the majority of patients, and always by the ninth month. There is a rapid enlargement during the first year.

PHYSICAL EXAMINATION

Skin Lesions

TYPE Nodule, 1.0 to 8.0 cm

COLOR The superficial angioma (strawberry mark) is bright red (Figures 120, 122, and 123); the deeper angioma (cavernous type) is purple and lobulated (Figure 121).

PALPATION Soft or moderately firm, depending on the proportionate amount of superficial or deep angiomatous elements

DISTRIBUTION Localized or extending over an entire region (e.g., cheek)

SITES OF PREDILECTION Face, trunk, legs, oral and vaginal mucous membrane

DIFFERENTIAL DIAGNOSIS

The distinction between a *strawberry mark* and a *cavernous angioma* is based on color and depth. Mixed angiomas (both superficial and deep) may occur.

DERMATOPATHOLOGY

Site Dermis and/or subcutaneous tissue
Process Proliferation of endothelial cells in varying amounts: There is more endothelial proliferation in the superficial type, and in the deep angiomas there is little or no endothelial proliferation.

COURSE AND PROGNOSIS

The strawberry mark type spontaneously involutes by the fifth year, with some few percent disappearing only by age 10. There is virtually no residual skin change at the site in most lesions (80 percent); in a significant percent, therefore, there is residual atrophy, depigmentation, and infiltration. Deep angiomatous nevi may not involute in over 40 percent of lesions, especially those lesions that occur on the mucous membrane.

TREATMENT

It is impossible to generalize, and each lesion must be judged individually regarding the decision to treat or not to treat and the selection of a treatment mode. Some options include surgical excision, systemic corticosteroids, sclerosing solutions, and liquid-nitrogen cryosurgery.

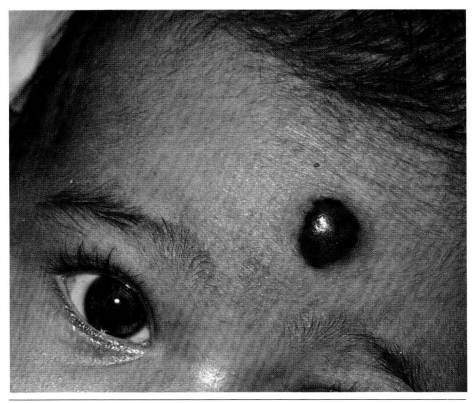

120 Strawberry nevus

Patient Profile   Three-month-old girl

History   Since birth, several red-purplish lesions on the forehead, right shoulder, in right groin, and on the tongue

Physical Examination   Elevated cherry-sized, red nodular tumor on the forehead, with smooth surface

Treatment   None. Spontaneous resolution is expected in 2 to 6 years. Regular supervision and photography to check rate of involution and to reassure the parents.

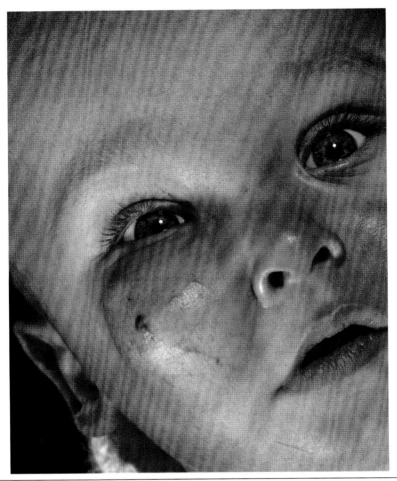

121 Cavernous hemangioma (subcutaneous type)

Patient Profile *Six-month-old girl*

History *Since birth, a large swelling on the right cheek. Until recently the tumor had steadily increased, but now growth has ceased.*

Physical Examination *Large, soft, semiglobular swelling with smooth surface. The color ranges from pale to purple. Some telangiectases are present. In the center is a small hemangioma. The tumor mass is also palpable on the inner side of the cheek. The eye split is slightly narrowed, but vision is not reduced.*

Laboratory and Special Examinations *No hematologic, ophthalmologic, or neurologic abnormalities*

Treatment *At the age of 8 years the tumor had entirely disappeared without residual scarring or discolorations.*

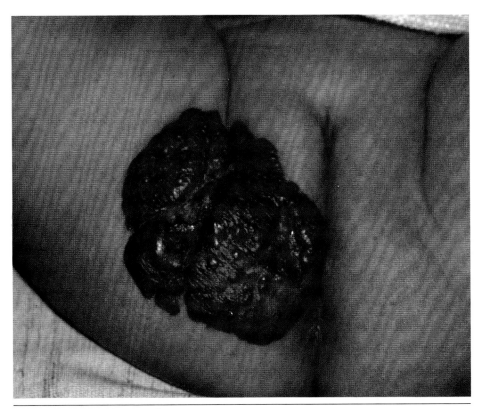

122 Cavernous hemangioma
Strawberry nevus

Patient Profile *Five-month-old girl*

History *Since birth, a large red tumor between right groin and vulva. Rapid growth, that now seems to have stopped. For 4 weeks, spontaneous ulceration without bleeding.*

Physical Examination *Large, approximately 15-mm thick, red-purplish tumor with sharp margin. Two ulcers are present. The underlying skin seems uninvolved. The surface of the left basal area shows a faint pale color, indicative of an initial spontaneous resolution.*

Laboratory and Special Examinations *Thrombocytes are normal.*

Treatment *No therapy. Course: see Figure 123*

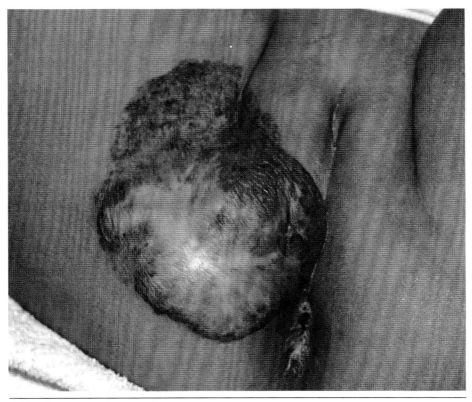

123   Cavernous hemangioma

Same child as in Figure 122, 8 months later. Impressive spontaneous resolution. Usually it takes much more time to achieve such an improvement. At the age of 3 years the tumor completely disappeared, leaving only mild atrophic changes and some hypo- and hypermelanosis.

Pyogenic Granuloma (Granuloma Telangiectaticum)

Pyogenic granuloma is a rapidly developing, bright red or violaceous or brown-black nodule that may be confused with malignant melanoma.

EPIDEMIOLOGY

Age Usually in children or persons under 30
Sex Equal incidence in males and females

HISTORY

Duration of Lesions Weeks
Skin Symptoms None; recurrent bleeding from the lesion may occur

PHYSICAL EXAMINATION

Skin Lesions See Figure 124.
TYPE Nodule with smooth or warty surface with or without crusts or erosions
COLOR Bright red, dusky red, violaceous, brown-black
SIZE AND SHAPE Less than 1.5 cm; usually lesion is pedunculated or sessile
DISTRIBUTION Isolated single lesion
SITES OF PREDILECTION Fingers, lips, mouth, trunk, toes

DIFFERENTIAL DIAGNOSIS

Malignant melanoma (especially amelanotic), *squamous cell carcinoma, glomus tumor*

DERMATOPATHOLOGY

Site Dermis with secondary epidermal involvement
Process Proliferation of capillaries with prominent endothelial cells embedded in edematous, gelatinous stromata

COURSE AND PROGNOSIS

Lesion does not spontaneously disappear and must be removed for a histologic diagnosis and treatment.

TREATMENT

Electrocautery, after removing tissue for histology.
Laser treatment is also effective, especially with the tunable dye laser.

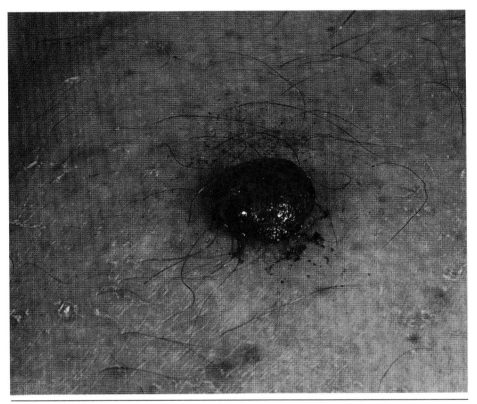

124 Granuloma pyogenicum
Granuloma telangiectaticum

Patient Profile Twenty-seven-year-old male

History For 2 weeks, rapidly increasing, friable, easily bleeding tumor on the shoulder. No pre-existing lesion or injury.

Physical Examination Nodular tumor, about 8 mm in diameter, sharply demarcated, erosive, partly hemorrhagic surface. The base is slightly constricted.

Differential Diagnosis Polyposis of granulation tissue, melanoma, hemangioma

Laboratory and Special Examinations Histology: atrophy of epidermis; dermis contains edematous and fibrous matrix, many newly formed blood vessels, and a marked inflammatory cellular infiltrate.

Clues Rapid development, polypoid or nodular appearance, and bleeding easily

Treatment Electrodesiccation under local anesthesia

XVIII

Premalignant and

Malignant Lesions

Epidermis
Melanocytes
Lymphoreticular Cells
Paget's Disease of the Nipple

Solar Keratosis (Actinic Keratosis)

These single or multiple, discrete, dry, rough, adherent scaly lesions occur on the habitually sun-exposed skin of adults.

EPIDEMIOLOGY AND ETIOLOGY

Age Middle age, although in Australia solar keratosis may occur in persons under 30
Sex More common in males
Race Skin Phototypes (SPT) I, II, and III (see Appendix D), rare in SPT IV, and almost never in blacks or East Indians
Occupation Outdoor workers (especially farmers, ranchers, sailors) and outdoor sportspersons (tennis, golf, mountain climbing, deep-sea fishing)

HISTORY

Duration of Lesions Months
Skin Symptoms Some lesions may be tender.

PHYSICAL EXAMINATION
Skin Lesions

TYPE

Adherent hyperkeratotic scale (Figure 125), which is removed with difficulty and pain
May be nodular

COLOR Skin-colored, yellow-brown, or brown; often there is a reddish tinge
PALPATION Rough, like coarse sandpaper (see Figure 125)
SIZE AND SHAPE Most commonly less than 1.0 cm; oval or round
DISTRIBUTION Isolated single lesion or scattered discrete lesions
SITES OF PREDILECTION Face (forehead, nose, cheeks, temples, vermilion border lower lip), ears (males), neck (sides), forearms and hands (dorsa)

DIFFERENTIAL DIAGNOSIS

Flat solar keratoses, especially red, may be confused with *discoid lupus erythematosus*. Biopsy is necessary.

DERMATOPATHOLOGY

Site Epidermis
Process Proliferative and neoplastic. Large bright-staining keratinocytes, with mild to moderate pleomorphism, parakeratosis, and atypical (dyskeratotic) keratinocytes

PATHOPHYSIOLOGY

Prolonged and repeated solar exposure in susceptible persons (Skin Types I, II, III) leads to cumulative damage to keratinocytes by the action of ultraviolet radiant energy, principally, if not exclusively, UVB (290 to 320 nm).

COURSE AND PROGNOSIS

Solar keratoses may spontaneously disappear, but in general they remain for years. The actual incidence of squamous cell carcinoma in preexisting solar keratoses is unknown.

TREATMENT AND PREVENTIVE MEASURES

Most solar keratoses react to local application to the lesion of 5% 5-fluorouracil cream over a period of several days and then disappear, but this often leads to depigmented spots. Short exposures to liquid nitrogen followed in 3 days by topical application of 5% 5-fluorouracil cream is most effective and avoids depigmented areas that occur when therapeutic exposures of liquid nitrogen are used alone.
Nodular lesions should be excised.
Prevention is afforded by use of highly effective UVB/UVA sunscreens, which should be applied daily to the face and ears during the summer in northern latitudes for Skin Types I and II and for those Skin Type III persons who obtain prolonged sunlight exposures.
Cryotherapy is also very effective.

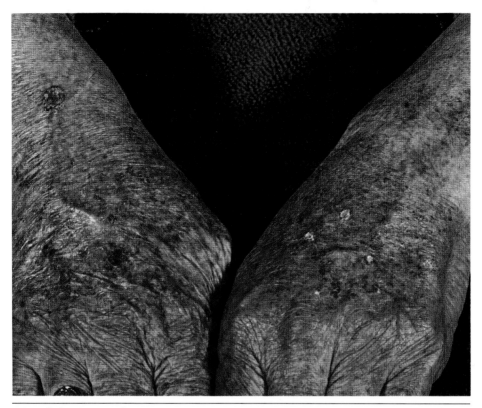

125 Solar keratosis
Actinic keratosis
Senile keratosis

Patient Profile Seventy-one-year-old retired fisherman

History For 2 years, on the backs of the hands, several small "crusts," bleeding easily after removal and recurring rapidly

Physical Examination The skin is atrophic, shows delicate wrinkling, several brown macules and small white-keratotic patches, 2 to 4 mm in size, partly surrounded by a narrow erythematous zone. No definite induration.

Differential Diagnosis Bowen's disease, incipient squamous cell carcinoma, cutaneous horns, lentigo simplex

Laboratory and Special Examinations Histology: hyperkeratosis, atrophy of epidermis, disorderly arrangement and occasional atypicality of prickle cells, and individual cell dyskeratosis. No invasive growth.

Clues Sun-damaged atrophic skin with small adherent keratotic patches

Treatment Cleared with 5% fluorouracil ointment for 14 days. Two resistant lesions were treated with liquid nitrogen.

Chronic x-ray dermatitis is defined as irreversible skin changes resulting from brief or prolonged, intense, repeated exposure to radiation of more than 1500 to 2000 rads.

TYPE OF EXPOSURE

Result of therapy (for cancer, acne, psoriasis), accidental (physician, dentist)

HISTORY

Duration of Lesions Months to years
Skin Symptoms Dryness, lack of sweating

PHYSICAL EXAMINATION

Skin Lesions See Figure 126

TYPE

Atrophy, with telangiectasia
Alopecia (permanent)
Papules, hyperkeratotic, "warty"
Hypopigmentation (circumscribed spotty)
Hyperpigmentation
Ulcers, indolent, painful

SHAPE

Sharp, rectangular, square (when result of therapy)
Diffuse involvement (when result of prolonged repeated exposures)

DISTRIBUTION

Hands and fingers (in professional personnel, dentists, or physicians)
Any site of previous therapy with ionizing radiation

Nails Longitudinal striations

DERMATOPATHOLOGY

Site Epidermis and dermis

1. Atrophy of epidermis, with loss of hair follicles, sebaceous glands, and alteration of sweat glands
2. Hyalinization, loss of nuclei, fusion of collagen and elastic tissue
3. Vessel changes including telangiectactic dilatation and fibrous thickening of the arterial walls

COURSE, PROGNOSIS, AND TREATMENT

Changes are permanent, and aggressive squamous cell carcinoma may develop. The area should be excised and grafted, if possible, or if mild to moderate damage, carefully followed for malignancy.

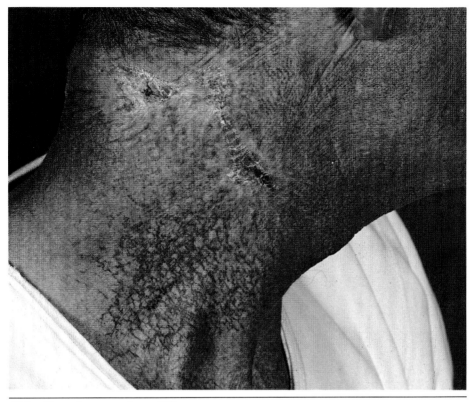

126   Chronic x-ray dermatitis

Patient Profile   *Fifty-year-old male*

History   *For 4 years, thinning and redness of right side of neck, and for 6 months, a scaling crusted area just below the scalp (see arrow) that does not heal. Received 10 years earlier, x-ray therapy (dose and quality remained unknown) for tuberculosis of skin and lymph nodes. Later on, treated with oral isonicotinic acid hydrazide (INH) for 3 years.*

Physical Examination   *The right side of the neck shows many telangiectases with a reticular pattern. The skin is atrophic. Near the scalp is a scaling crusted patch; after removal of this crust a superficial ulcer became apparent. Just below the lower mandibula is a somewhat linear, erythematous, slightly indurated scaling lesion.*

Laboratory and Special Examinations   *Biopsies from crusted area and linear lesion: no signs of tuberculosis or malignancy.*

Clues   *History of x-ray treatment, abundant telangiectases, atrophy, ulcer, histopathology*

Treatment   *The ulcerating lesion did not respond to various ointments and was slowly progressive. Ultimately excision and grafting gave a satisfactory result.*

Oral Leukoplakia

Leukoplakia "is a white patch or plaque that cannot be characterized clinically or pathologically as any other disease." (Definition of World Health Organization's Collaborating Centre for Oral Precancerous Lesions, 1978)

EPIDEMIOLOGY

Age Forty to seventy years
Sex Males, rarely in females
Race Common in fair-skinned persons

HISTORY

Duration of Lesions Years
Skin Symptoms None

PHYSICAL EXAMINATION

Mucous Membrane Lesions

TYPE Small or large plaque; homogeneous or "speckled" ulceration may be present
COLOR Gray-white
PALPATION Moderately rough or leathery
SHAPE AND SIZE Angular. Size varies from small (2.0 cm) to very large (4.0 cm) plaque on the hard palate
SITES OF PREDILECTION Buccal mucosa (Figure 127), retrocommissural mucosa, tongue, hard palate, sublingual region, and gingiva

DIFFERENTIAL DIAGNOSIS

Lichen planus (see Figure 37), *oral hairy leukoplakia* occurring in HIV-infected individuals

DERMATOPATHOLOGY

Site Epidermis
Process Neoplastic. Dysplasia of keratinocytes with keratinization of single cells, abnormal mitosis, increased nuclear/cytoplasmic ratio, cell and nuclear pleomorphism, enlarged and/or multiple nucleoli

PATHOPHYSIOLOGY

A premalignant lesion arising from chronic irritation or inflammation. Certain types carry a high risk for developing malignancy: (1) leukoplakia with candidiasis, (2) leukoplakia that is speckled (with gray and white patches) rather than homogeneous, (3) in certain sites—floor of the mouth and central surface of the tongue. Pipe and cigar smoking produces *leukokeratosis nicotina palati,* which rarely becomes malignant.

TREATMENT

Surgical excision or cryotherapy

Leukoplakia type lesions on the lip respond very well to topical vitamin-A acid, 0.05% cream

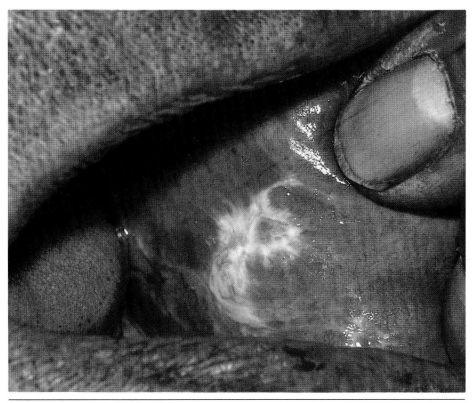

127 Leukoplakia of the mouth

Patient Profile Fifty-five-year-old male

History For 2 years, a slowly progressive, asymptomatic white plaque on the buccal mucosa. Smokes four cigars a day. No other skin lesions

Physical Examination On the inner side of the left cheek is a white, slightly elevated plaque with an irregular margin and firm consistency. The surface is rough. An improperly fitted denture presses against the lesion.

Differential Diagnosis Candidiasis, lichen planus of the mouth

Laboratory and Special Examinations Histology: marked hyperkeratosis, acanthosis with occasional atypicality of cells, basal layer intact. Direct microscopy and culture for Candida: negative.

Clues White, firm, keratotic plaque on mucosa

Treatment Excision of the lesion by oral surgeon. Correction of the denture plate. Advice to not smoke.

Basal Cell Carcinoma (Noduloulcerative)

Basal cell carcinoma, the most common form of skin cancer, occurs as an isolated hard papule or nodule on the face; ulceration and invasion frequently occur but metastasis is very rare.

EPIDEMIOLOGY AND ETIOLOGY

Age Over 40 years
Sex Males have a somewhat higher incidence than females.
Incidence
539:100,000 (Dallas)
174:100,000 (Iowa)
Race Very rare in pigmented peoples of all races
Predisposing Factors More common in Skin Phototypes I and II and in white persons of any skin type who obtain prolonged intensive insolation (sailors, farmers, telephone repairmen, professional fishermen, etc.). Persons living in Australia or southern United States. Other etiologic agents are inorganic trivalent arsenic, exposure to ionizing radiation, genetic (basal cell nevus syndrome).
Significance In the United States there are over 400,000 new white patients with nonmelanoma skin cancer, and in the Southwest the incidence approaches 1000 per 100,000 population. This is directly related to the duration and intensity of solar ultraviolet radiation.

HISTORY

Duration of Lesions Slow-growing; months, even years
Skin Symptoms Usually asymptomatic unless ulceration occurs and then there is frequently bleeding

PHYSICAL EXAMINATION

Skin Lesions

TYPE

Papule or nodule. Translucent or pearly and shiny.
Ulcer (often covered with a crust) may occur in the center of the nodule (Figures 128 and 129); when the crust is removed, bleeding occurs.

COLOR Pink or red; telangiectasia observed with a hand lens
PALPATION The lesion is hard, not firm.
SHAPE Round, oval, often umbilicated (Figures 128 and 129)
DISTRIBUTION Isolated lesion; exposed areas of the head (especially central part of the face)

DIFFERENTIAL DIAGNOSIS

Dermal melanocytic nevi (Figure 116) may be almost impossible to distinguish from papular or nodular type basal cell carcinoma (Figure 130); biopsy is necessary. For proper examination the patient should be on an examination table and the physician viewing the face with a strong light and using a hand lens. Basal cell carcinoma is often multiple and early lesions may be missed.

DERMATOPATHOLOGY

Site Epidermis and dermis
Process Neoplastic. Invading masses of basal cell carcinoma cells (large, oval, elongated nucleus, staining deep blueblack with hematoxylin) with little anaplasia and no abnormal mitoses

TREATMENT AND PROGNOSIS

Biopsy of all suspected tumors is essential. The choice of treatment depends on the *type of basal cell carcinoma* (noduloulcerative vs. fibrosing vs. superficial) and the *location* (lesions around the nose, eyes, and ears should have definitive therapy: surgical excision, Mohs surgery, or radiotherapy); cryotherapy and electrocautery are acceptable modalities for lesions on the trunk or upper extremities. If these guidelines are followed, the cure rate is 95 percent.

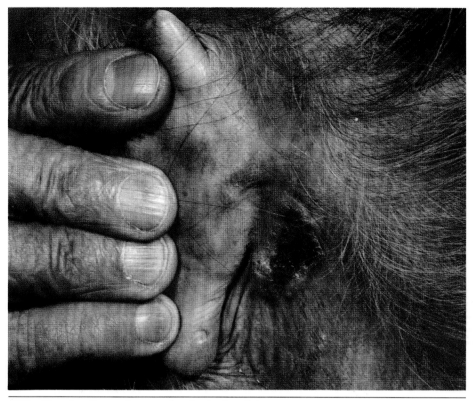

128　Basal cell carcinoma, "rodent ulcer" type

Patient Profile　Sixty-five-year-old female

History　For 6 months, a gradually enlarging ulceration behind the left ear, caused (according to patient) by irritation from spectacles

Physical Examination　A solitary ulcer with firm elevated border and an occasional crust, diameter 2.5 cm

Dermatopathology　Nests and strands of the dark-staining nonkeratinizing basal cells arising from the epidermis and invading into the dermis

Clues　Typical firm, rolled, translucent border with telangiectasia; biopsy confirmation

Significance　An ulcer that does not heal in a month must be suspected of malignancy until proved otherwise by biopsy.

COURSE AND FOLLOW-UP

All patients to be followed at 6-month intervals for the first 2 years and then yearly if there are no new lesions

Lesions in high-risk areas (nasolabial folds, postauricular, or periorbital) to be followed every 6 months for 3 years

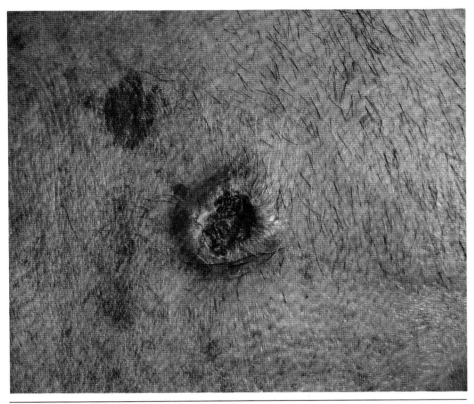

129 Basal cell carcinoma, "rodent ulcer" type

Patient Profile Fifty-eight-year-old gardener

History For 9 months, an ulceration on the left temple

Physical Examination A solitary ulceration, diameter 2 cm, surrounded by a whitish, translucent, elevated border, with an erythematous margin and telangiectases. Also signs of solar damage: irregular pigmentation and depigmentation, telangiectases, and a round brown macule.

Dermatopathology Strands of darkly stained cells arise from the epidermis; isles of similar cells with marginal palisading are present in the cutis.

Clues Firm, translucent, rolled border; histopathology

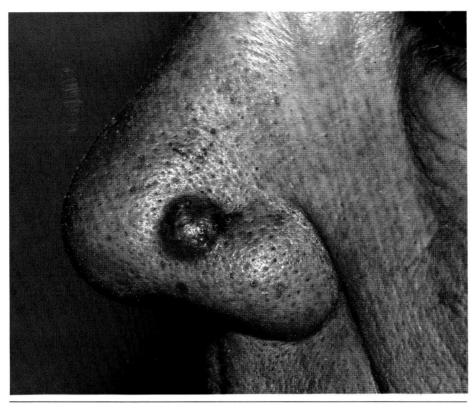

130　Basal cell carcinoma, nodular type

Patient Profile　Fifty-eight-year-old male bricklayer

History　For 3 months, a slowly growing tumor on left ala of the nose

Physical Examination　Firm, 1.5-cm nodule with telangiectases

Differential Diagnosis　Dermal melanocytic nevus

Dermatopathology　Nests of small cells in the dermis with peripheral palisading, connected in a few places by strands with the epidermis: basal cell carcinoma.

Clues　History, firm translucent nodule with telangiectases, dermatopathology

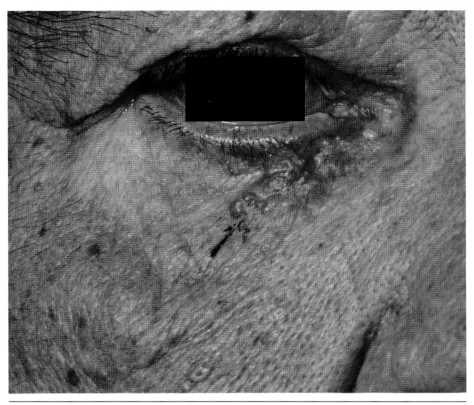

131 Basal cell carcinoma, nodular type

Patient Profile Eighty-two-year-old female homemaker

History For 10 years, an asymptomatic eruption under right eye that started as a "wart." This was once treated with electrocoagulation.

Physical Examination Disseminated, firm, skin-colored, translucent nodules over an area of 7 to 20 mm, partly coalescent

Dermatopathology Atrophic epidermis; in the dermis, areas of hyperchromatic epithelial cells occasionally polymorphous; a rare mitosis, marginal palisading

Clues Dermatopathology; typical firm, translucent papules and nodules with telangiectases

Treatment Superficial x-ray

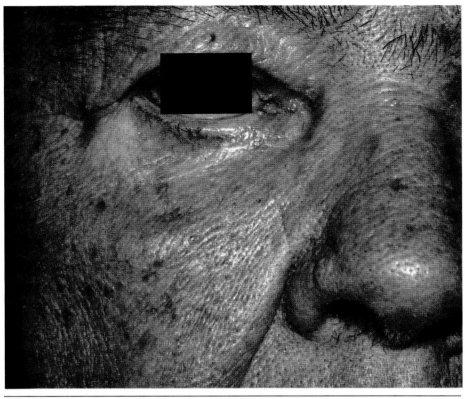

132 Basal cell carcinoma, nodular type

Result of the irradiation after 8 months (same patient as in Figure 131)

Basal Cell Carcinoma (Pigmented)

It is virtually impossible to diagnose this pigmented basal cell on clinical examination alone as it mimics nodular malignant melanoma. If in doubt (which one always is), a simple excision will establish the diagnosis. If it is, in fact, a nodular malignant melanoma, a wide reexcision must be done.

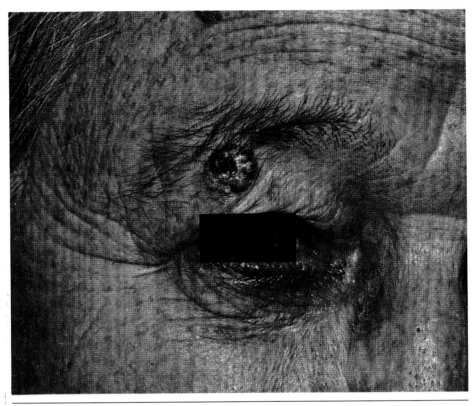

133 Basal cell carcinoma, pigmented type

Patient Profile *Seventy-six-year-old female homemaker*

History *For 2 years, a slowly growing, occasionally bleeding tumor on right upper eyelid*

Physical Examination *On right upper eyelid, a firm nodule, 2.5 × 2.5 cm, irregular surface, ulceration in center. Color: brownish black, translucent.*

Differential Diagnosis *Nodular malignant melanoma*

Dermatopathology *Thin atrophic epidermis; in the dermis, large areas consisting of hyperchromatic cells with peripheral palisading. A number of the basal cells contain a brown pigment. This pigment is also densely scattered in the dermis between a massive cellular infiltration of the stroma with lymphocytes and plasma cells.*

Clues *Hard to palpation; translucent areas with telangiectasia; dermatopathology*

Basal Cell Carcinoma (Fibrosing Type)

The typical hard, rolled, translucent border is distinctive for basal cell carcinoma. These lesions are deceptive in their breadth and depth and are best managed with radiation therapy or "fresh tissue" (Mohs) surgery.

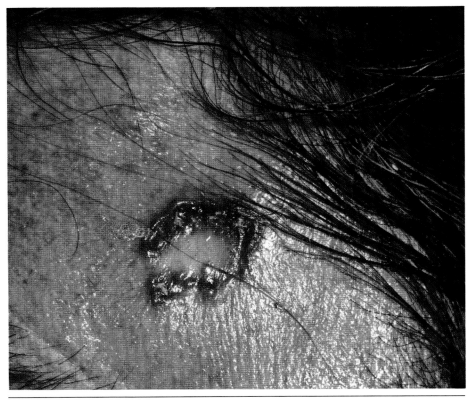

134 Basal cell carcinoma, cicatrizing type

Patient Profile Sixty-eight-year-old female homemaker

History Three years

Physical Examination An elevated, erythematous, solitary tumor of hard consistency; in some places, a "pearly border." At the center: boardlike skin without the normal skin markings.

Dermatopathology From an atrophic epidermis, buds and strands of hyperchromatic basal cells grow into the dermis.

Clues Pearly hard border with a central firm white area; dermatopathology

Basal Cell Carcinoma (Superficial Type)

This type of basal cell carcinoma presents a problem in differential diagnosis, closely simulating a localized plaque of eczema or psoriasis. A definitive clinical diagnosis can be made by careful examination of the lesion using a hand lens, which reveals a pathognomonic "threadlike" translucent border (see arrow, Figure 135). Superficial basal cell carcinoma virtually never occurs on the face, but on the trunk.

TREATMENT

Treatment of superficial basal cell carcinoma should be definitive, and therefore topical fluorouracil should not be used as recurrences almost always occur. Cryotherapy is ideal for smaller lesions (less than 5.0 cm), while x-radiation is best for large lesions.

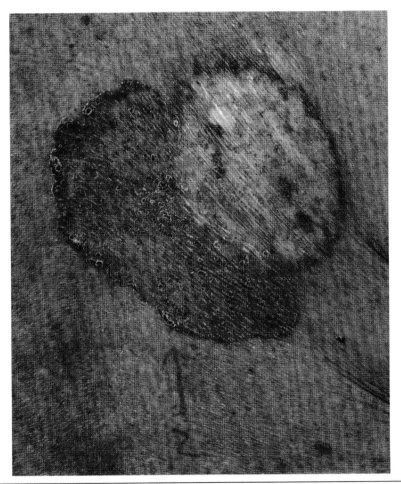

135 Basal cell carcinoma, multicentric superficial type

Patient Profile Sixty-three-year-old female homemaker

History Five years ago, a spot on the back was irradiated, which produced a scar; now, next to this irradiated spot, an itching, slowly growing lesion.

Physical Examination On the back, a plaque of 6 × 5 cm merging with an atrophic macule. The plaque shows a reticular red infiltration with a slightly elevated, firm, scaling border with a pearl-like aspect. The right-hand lesion is white, atrophic, with telangiectases and a red border.

Differential Diagnosis Psoriasis, eczema, tinea corporis

Dermatopathology Basal cell carcinoma

Clues Atrophy, depigmentation, and telangiectases (x-ray); "threadlike" rolled border; biopsy confirmation

Squamous Cell Carcinoma (SCC)

This tumor usually arises from keratinocytes that have been damaged by exogenous agents acting as carcinogens—sunlight, x-rays, arsenic ingestion. In its most common form it is a tumor arising on the sun-exposed areas in older people.

EPIDEMIOLOGY AND ETIOLOGY

Age Over fifty-five
Sex Males predominate except for lower legs, where women have a higher incidence
Race Highest incidence in Skin Phototype I and II persons living in areas of high insolation (see Appendix D)
Other Predisposing Factors Smoking (especially pipe and cigar), industrial carcinogens (tars and oils), chronic ulcers, old burn scars, discoid lupus erythematosus

HISTORY

Duration of Lesions Insidious, over months
Skin Symptoms None unless ulcerated

PHYSICAL EXAMINATION

Skin Lesions

TYPE

Indurated papule, plaque, or nodule (see Figures 136 and 138)
Adherent keratotic scale, often eroded, crusted, and ulcerated (see Figures 136 and 138)

COLOR Erythematous
PALPATION *Hard* (the most unique feature of SCC); may be fixed to structure below
SHAPE Polygonal, oval, round, umbilicated

DISTRIBUTION

Isolated lesion or a few scattered discrete lesions
Exposed areas (head, neck, dorsa of hands, forearms, legs in females, lips (Figure 136), tip of ear (Figure 138)

Miscellaneous Physical Findings Regional lymphadenopathy (35 percent in SCC arising in mouth or on lip)

DIFFERENTIAL DIAGNOSIS

Any isolated, keratotic, eroded, ulcerating papule, plaque, or nodule that persists more than 1 month is carcinoma until proved otherwise.

DERMATOPATHOLOGY

Site Epidermis, dermis, subcutaneous tissue
Process Anaplastic proliferation. Invasive strands of atypical cells: irregular shape and size, enlarged nuclei, abnormal mitoses. Varying degrees of keratinization

TREATMENT

The selection of treatment depends on the *size, shape,* and *localization of the tumor* and the *predisposing factors* (e.g., whether arising in radiation dermatitis or in chronic dermatoheliosis or on the lip). The choice of therapy should be made by a dermatologist in collaboration with a radiation therapist and a surgeon.
Squamous cell carcinoma arising on the dorsum of the hand (see Figure 137) should be treated by excision and grafting.

PROGNOSIS

The overall 5-year remission rate is 90 percent, including SCC of the lip. The incidence of metastasis of SCC is not as high. Squamous cell carcinoma arising in a solar keratosis has a low potential for metastasis (3 percent), while SCC arising in radiation dermatitis, tar keratosis, or old burn scars is more likely to metastasize (20 to 26 percent).

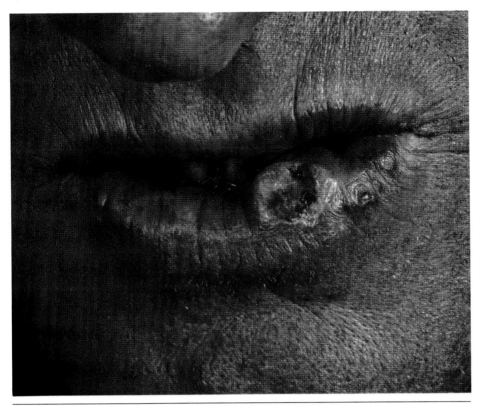

136 Squamous cell carcinoma

Patient Profile *Fifty-one-year-old florist*

History *For 6 months, a swelling on the left side of lower lip, occasional bleeding; no recent increase in size*

Physical Examination *An elevated ulcerating nodule on the left lower lip. No lymphadenopathy.*

Dermatopathology *Growth in the dermis of irregular epithelial, principally squamous, cells with numerous mitoses; individual cell keratinization and horn cysts, surrounded by an inflammatory infiltration*

Clues *Hard nodule in a typical location*

Treatment *Wide wedge-shaped excision of the ulcerating tumor. No recurrence after 5 years.*

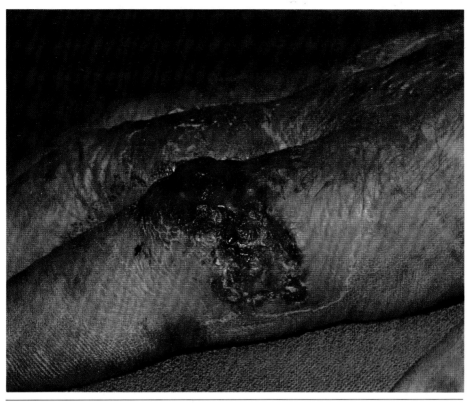

137 Squamous cell carcinoma

Patient Profile *Eighty-three-year-old retired fisherman*

History *For 10 years, ulcerations on finger II of the left hand, which were tended by the patient in a very unhygienic way*

Physical Examination *Ulcerations, 1.5 × 2 cm, with a serpiginous elevated border and a red granulating floor. (On the dorsal side of the phalanx of finger III, redness with a scaling border.) The ulcer was freely movable in relation to the bone. No enlargement of regional lymph nodes.*

Differential Diagnosis *Basal cell carcinoma*

Dermatopathology *The whole skin is invaded by fields of well-differentiated epithelial cells which form pearls, polymorphous nuclei, and a few mitoses. Fields of necrosis in the center of the tumor.*

Clues *Dermatopathology and clinical aspect*

Treatment *Surgical. During the operation the tumor mass proved to have grown into the tendons; this necessitated an amputation.*

Prognosis *Uneventful healing of the amputation wound; no metastases during the lifetime of patient, who died 2 years later from a cerebrovascular accident*

Significance *Every chronic ulceration is suspect for malignancy. On the hand, most malignancies are squamous cell carcinomas.*

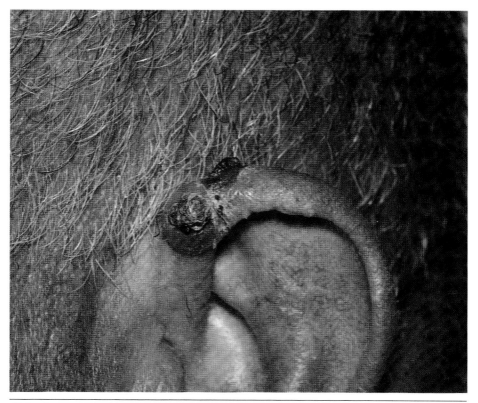

138 Squamous cell carcinoma

Patient Profile Sixty-year-old male florist

History For 2 years, a horny growth on the left helix. Had been repeatedly treated with curettage elsewhere.

Physical Examination On the proximal upper part of the helix, a firm red round tumor, 1.4 cm in diameter, within the center a horny crust. Moreover, more distal on the top of the helix, a glassy papule, 0.8 cm in diameter, with a horn plug. The tumor is asymptomatic.

Differential Diagnosis Basal cell carcinoma, chondrodermatitis nodularis helicis

Dermatopathology Punch biopsies from both tumors essentially the same result: in the dermis, fields of epithelial cells with individual cell keratinization, irregular cell differentiation, many mitoses, and a rare giant nucleus.

Clues Dermatopathology and clinical aspect

Treatment Excision by a plastic surgeon and reconstruction of the concha

Prognosis and Significance No recurrence after 5 years. In other areas several actinic keratoses.

Lentigo Maligna and Lentigo Maligna Melanoma

Lentigo maligna (LM), unlike the relatively uniform brown macules of solar lentigo, develops, over time, variations of brown color (tan, dark brown, even black) and irregularly irregular borders. Focal areas of the lesions become raised (papular), and this signals invasion into the dermis; it is then called lentigo maligna melanoma (LMM).

EPIDEMIOLOGY AND ETIOLOGY

Age Median age is 70.
Sex Equal sex ratio
Race Very rare in Asians, American Indians, blacks, and Skin Phototype (SPT) IV Caucasians. Highest incidence in SPT I to III Caucasians
Predisposing Factors Outdoor workers, much like nonmelanoma skin cancer

PHYSICAL EXAMINATION

Skin Lesions

TYPE (See Figure 139)

Lentigo maligna Two to 20 cm, exclusively macular
Lentigo maligna melanoma Focal areas of papules or nodules

COLOR Variations in hue from tan to black, stippled with black, and a haphazard network of black on a background of tan or brown (Figure 139). Gray areas indicate regression (northeast border in Figure 139).
SHAPE *Irregularly irregular borders, often with a notch* (see Figure 139)
DISTRIBUTION Usually isolated single lesion on the exposed areas: forehead, nose, cheeks, neck, forearms, and dorsa of hands (see page 390)

DERMATOPATHOLOGY

See Appendix F, Figure F-1.

TREATMENT AND PROGNOSIS

See Appendix F, pages 391–392.
For Recommendations for the Management of Pigmented Lesions to Facilitate Early Diagnosis of Malignant Melanomas, see Appendix F, page 366.

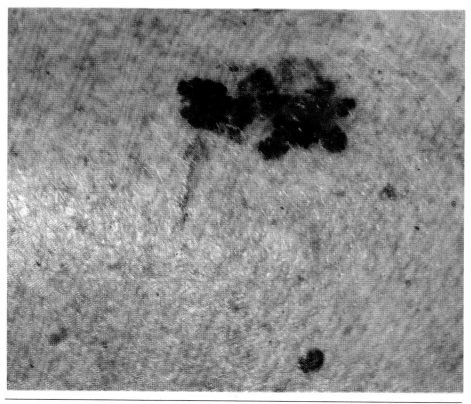

139 Lentigo maligna melanoma

Patient Profile Seventy-two-year-old bulb grower

History For 6 months, a "spot" on the left shoulder

Physical Examination On the left shoulder, a serpiginous macule comprised of two different lesions: on the right the macule is variegated and brown-black; on the left side (arrow) the lesion is slightly elevated and almost exclusively black.

Differential Diagnosis Superficial spreading melanoma

Histopathology Lentigo maligna melanoma, level II, 0.44 mm in thickness

Superficial spreading melanoma (SSM) is the most frequently observed melanoma arising in the skin. It is a moderately slow-growing (1 to 7 years) pigmented plaque and appears in middle age but is being increasingly observed in young adults.

EPIDEMIOLOGY AND ETIOLOGY

Age   Median age is 47.
Sex   Equal sex ratio
Race   Highest incidence in Caucasians, Skin Phototypes I to III (see Appendix D)
Predisposing Factors   Superficial spreading melanoma is the "new" neoplasm of post World War II, as the incidence has increased sixfold since 1945. This increased incidence is observed mostly in young professionals working indoors who receive intermittent intense sun exposure ("weekenders") or "charter flight" people from the northern latitudes who sun near the equator during the winter. Fifty percent or more of SSM arise in preexisting nevi (see pages 347 and 353). See Appendix F, pages 386 and 394.

PHYSICAL EXAMINATION

Skin Lesions

TYPE   Flattened papule → plaque, then developing one or more nodules (see Figure 140)
COLOR   Marked, haphazard variegation: brown, black, pink, red, and whitish gray (sites of regression) (see Figure 140)
SHAPE AND SIZE   Arciform, *irregularly irregular border* and *often a notch;* mean diameter 2.0 cm, some lesions as small as 0.2 cm

DISTRIBUTION

Isolated single lesions, rarely multiple primaries
Sites of origin (see page 390)

Upper back (males and females)
Face and lower legs (females)
Anterior trunk and legs (males)
Covered areas spared (bathing suit area in females, bathing trunk area in males)

DIAGNOSIS OF EARLY MELANOMA

See Appendix F, pages 386 and 388.

DERMATOPATHOLOGY

See Appendix F, Figure F-2

PATHOPHYSIOLOGY

Superficial spreading melanoma is the most frequently observed melanoma of all types and the rate of increase in incidence in recent years has paralleled that of lung cancer. The reasons are not clear, but there is increasing evidence for the role of solar radiation in the pathogenesis of SSM.

TREATMENT

See Appendix F, page 391.

PROGNOSIS

See Appendix F, page 392.

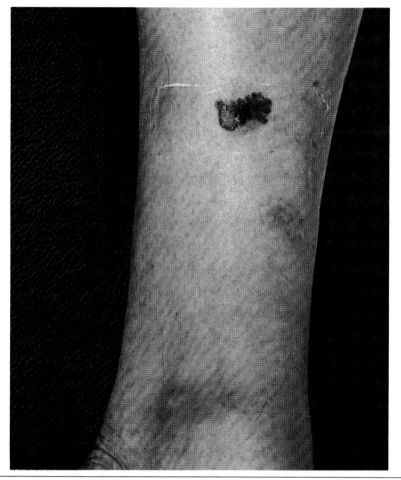

140 Superficial spreading melanoma

Patient Profile Seventy-three-year-old female

History According to the patient, there was "always" a spot on the left lower leg; lately a dark, occasionally bleeding, tumor has developed.

Physical Examination A black, firm, slightly elevated tumor, 1.1 × 1.4 cm in diameter, with a tiny blood crust is present in the center of a brown irregularly demarcated area 2.5 × 1.2 cm in diameter.

Differential Diagnosis Hemangioma

Histopathology Superficial spreading melanoma, level IV, 3.1 mm in thickness

Clues Clinical aspect and histopathology

Just as with lentigo maligna melanoma (LMM) or superficial spreading melanoma (SSM), this lesion arises from normal skin or from a preexisting congenital or acquired nevocellular nevus. However, there is little or no intraepidermal or "radial" growth as in LMM or SSM; rather, there is virtually only "vertical growth."

EPIDEMIOLOGY AND ETIOLOGY

Age Median age is 50.
Sex Same as for SSM
Race Same as for SSM
Predisposing Factors Same as for SSM

PHYSICAL EXAMINATION

Skin Lesions

TYPE Nodule (see Figure 141), noduloulcerative, thick plaque (rare)
COLOR Blue or blue-black, uniform color, pink (amelanotic) with traces of brown and black (see Figure 141)
SIZE AND SHAPE Polypoid, dome-shaped, 1.0 to 3.0 cm (see Figure 142)

DISTRIBUTION Same as superficial spreading melanoma (see also page 390)

DERMATOPATHOLOGY

See Appendix F, Figure F-3

TREATMENT

See Appendix F, page 391.

PROGNOSIS

See Appendix F, page 392.

Malignant Melanoma Arising in a Preexisting Nevocellular Nevus

The lifetime risk of developing a malignant melanoma in a *giant* congenital nevus cell nevus (GCNN) (so-called garment nevus or bathing-trunk nevus) is at least 6.3 percent, and these melanomas often appear before the age of *5 years.* Giant congenital nevus cell nevi are lesions that cover large areas of the body.

Based on the detection of congenital nevi in association with melanoma using histology and a careful history, there is a significantly increased risk for developing melanoma in persons with small congenital nevus cell nevi (SCNN). This risk is as high as 21-fold based on history, and three- to tenfold based on histology. Fifteen percent of 134 patients with primary cutaneous melanoma stated that the melanoma arose in a congenital nevus. Of 234 primary melanomas, 8.1 percent had nevus cell nevi with congenital features. The expected association of SCNN and melanoma is less than 1 in 171,000 based on chance alone. Therefore, all SCNN should be considered for prophylactic excision at puberty if there are no atypical features (variegated color and irregular borders); SCNN with atypical features should be excised immediately. (See Congenital Nevomelanocytic Nevus, page 296.)

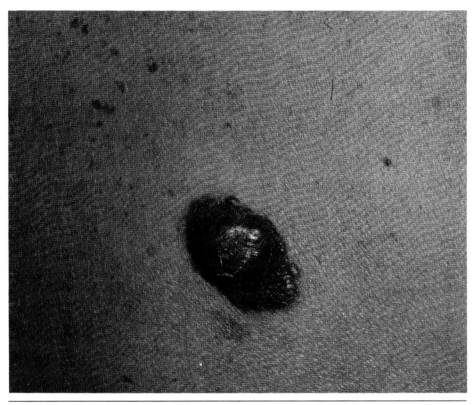

141 Nodular malignant melanoma

Patient Profile Twenty-nine-year-old female homemaker

History According to the patient, a mole had been present for a long time. A year ago she was injured by a seashell when lying on the beach. The center had grown and it bled occasionally.

Physical Examination Over the right scapula there is an oval, firm, sharply demarcated 3-cm tumor. At the margins the surface is papillomatous; in the center the tumor is more elevated and has a smooth surface and a glassy bluish-brown aspect. No regional lymphadenopathy.

Differential Diagnosis Pigmented basal cell carcinoma

Histopathology Nodular malignant melanoma, level V, 4.2 mm in thickness

Clues Histopathology and clinical aspect

Treatment and Course Excision and skin graft. Follow-up after a year was symptom-free. After 2 years, skin metastases appeared on the neck and thorax. The patient died 3 years after the first surgery.

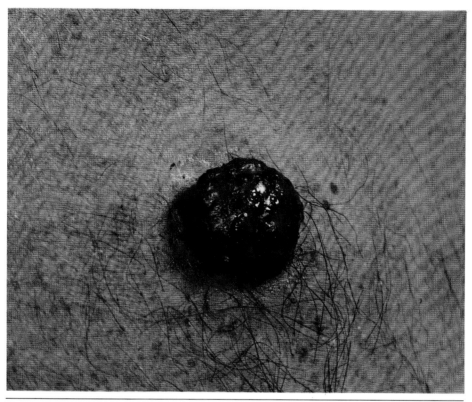

142 Nodular malignant melanoma

Patient Profile Fifty-one-year-old bricklayer

History A tumor on the back had been present for several years.

Physical Examination On the right scapula is a mushroom-shaped, partially red, otherwise black, firm tumor, round and sharply demarcated. Diameter: 1.5 cm; elevation above surrounding skin: 3 mm. In the right axilla, lymph nodes are palpable.

Differential Diagnosis Granuloma pyogenicum, hemangioma

Histopathology Nodular malignant melanoma, level III, 5.6 mm in thickness, with positive regional lymph nodes

Clues Histopathology and clinical aspect

Treatment and Course Excision of primary tumor and radical node dissection. In the following 2 years there were reoperations for metastases in axillary and inguinal lymph nodes and metastases of the abdominal wall. Chemotherapy, but patient died from cerebral metastases 3 years after the primary operation.

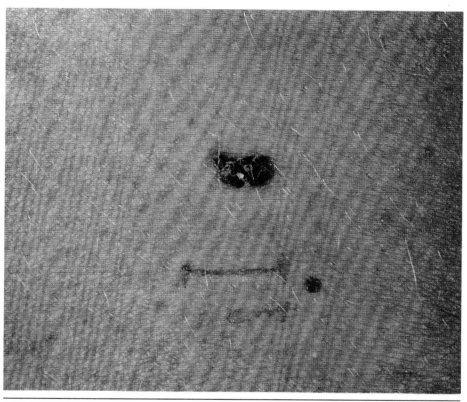

143   Hemangioma pseudomelanoticum

Patient Profile   Eighteen-year-old female

History   The patient stated that a mole had always been present on the thigh and lately the lesion bled.

Physical Examination   A brown-black, slightly elevated spot, 0.6 to 0.3 cm in diameter, with scales and crusts

Differential Diagnosis   Melanoma, thrombosed hemangioma

Histopathology   Excision biopsy: thrombosed capillary aneurysm.

Clue   Pathology

Significance   When a patient states that a mole that has been asymptomatic for a long time begins to bleed following trauma, it is highly suggestive of an incipient melanoma. This case illustrates that this is not necessarily so.

Mycosis Fungoides (Cutaneous T-Cell Lymphoma, CTCL)

Mycosis fungoides applies to T-cell lymphoma manifested first in the skin, but, as the neoplastic process involves the entire lymphoreticular system, the lymph nodes and internal organs become involved later in the course of the disease. CTCL is a malignancy of helper T cells.

EPIDEMIOLOGY AND ETIOLOGY

Age Fifty years (range, 5 to 70 years) years)
Sex Male/female ratio: 2 : 1
Incidence Two per 1,000,000 population. Accounts for 1 percent of deaths from lymphoma (about 200 deaths per year in the United States).
Etiology Human T-cell leukemia/lymphoma virus in some patients

HISTORY

Duration of Lesions Months to years, often preceded by nonspecific or false-negative diagnoses such as psoriasis, nummular dermatitis, and "large plaque" parapsoriasis
Skin Symptoms Pruritus, often intractable, but may be none
Constitutional Symptoms Fever (in late tumor stage)
Systems Review Negative except in late stages with visceral organ involvement

PHYSICAL EXAMINATION

Skin Lesions

TYPE

Plaques, scaling or not scaling, large (>3.0 cm) (see Figures 144 and 145), at first superficial, much like "eczema" or psoriasis, and later becoming thicker or "infiltrated"
Nodules and tumors with or without ulcers (see Figure 146)

COLOR Different shades of red
SHAPE Round, oval, arciform, annular, concentric, bizarre shapes (see Figure 144)
ARRANGEMENT Randomly distributed discrete plaques, nodules, and tumors, or diffuse involvement with erythroderma (Sézary's syndrome) and palmoplantar keratosis

DISTRIBUTION

Often spares exposed areas (in early stages)
No typical distribution pattern, random localization

Other Physical Findings Careful examination for lymphadenopathy

DIFFERENTIAL DIAGNOSIS

High index of suspicion is needed in patients with atypical or refractory psoriasis, eczema, and poikiloderma atrophicans vasculare. Repeated biopsies are necessary. Mycosis fungoides often mimics psoriasis in being a scaly plaque and disappearing with sunlight exposure.

LABORATORY AND SPECIAL STUDIES

Repeated and multiple (3) biopsies often necessary to finally establish the diagnosis

Dermatopathology

SITE Epidermis and dermis

1. Mycosis cells: T cells with hyperchromic, irregularly shaped nuclei. Mytoses vary from rare to frequent.

2. Microabscesses in the lower epidermis (containing "mycosis" cells).

3. Bandlike and patchy infiltrate in upper dermis of atypical lymphocytes (mycosis cells), and extending to skin appendages. Abnormal "T" cells can be identified by electron microscopy: typically convoluted nucleus.

4. Monoclonal-antibody techniques identify most mycosis cells as helper/inducer T cells.

Hematologic Eosinophilia, 6 to 12 percent, could increase to 50 percent. Abnormal circulating T cells (Sézary type) and increased white blood count (20,000). Bone marrow examination is not helpful.
Blood Chemistry Lactic dehydrogenase isoenzymes 1, 2, 3 increased in erythrodermic stage.
Chest X-Ray
Liver-Spleen Scan To identify any focal areas

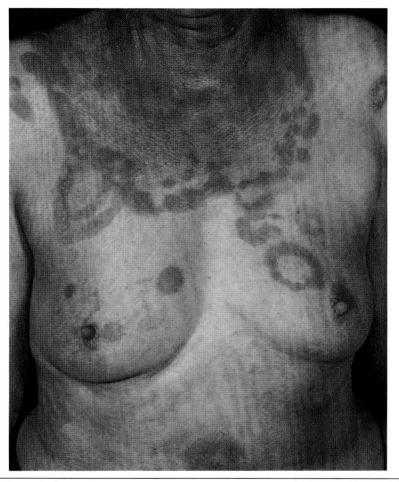

144   Mycosis fungoides

Patient Profile   Sixty-seven-year-old female homemaker

History   For 4 years, a red scaling eruption on the face, trunk, and extremities, which was diagnosed as an atypical psoriasis, responding poorly to corticosteroids and anthralin

Physical Examination   Annular, serpiginous, red scaling plaques on the trunk

Differential Diagnosis   Psoriasis

Histopathology   In the dermis, bandlike infiltration with mononuclear cells with cerebriform nuclei that penetrate into the epidermis

CAT Scan To search for retroperitoneal nodes in patients with extensive skin involvement, lymphadenopathy, or tumors in the skin

DIAGNOSIS

In the early stages the diagnosis of mycosis fungoides is a problem. Clinical lesions may be typical but histologic confirmation may not be possible for years despite repeated biopsies. One-μm thick sections may be helpful. For early diagnosis, cytophotometry (estimation of aneuploidy and polyploidy) and estimation of the indentation of pathologic cells (nucleocontour index) are helpful. Fresh tissue should be sent for analysis of cellular makeup by the use of monoclonal antibodies. Lymphadenopathy and the detection of abnormal circulating T cells in the blood appear to correlate well with *internal* organ involvement and surgical staging is not necessary. See TNM classification (Table).

COURSE AND PROGNOSIS

The course is quite unpredictable until a histologic diagnosis is made; i.e., a clinical diagnosis of suspicious mycosis fungoides (pre-mycosis fungoides) may be present for years. Once histologic diagnosis is made, the course of the disease varies with the source of the patient material studied: at the National Institutes of Health in the United States there was a median survival rate of 5 years from the time of the histologic diagnosis, while in England a less malignant course is seen; and, simi-larly, it would appear that, in office practice, there is a prolonged course (sometimes 10 to 15 years). After histologic diagnosis is made, everyone agrees that prognosis is much worse when (1) tumors are present (mean survival, 2.5 years), (2) there is lymphadenopathy (mean survival, 3 years), (3) more than 10 percent of the skin surface is involved with pre-tumor stage mycosis fungoides, and (4) there is a generalized erythroderma. Patients under 50 have twice the survival rate of patients over 60 years.

TREATMENT

In the pre-mycosis fungoides stage, in which the histologic diagnosis is not established, PUVA photochemotherapy is the least harmful effective treatment. For histologically proved plaque-stage disease with no lymphadenopathy and with no circulating abnormal T cells, PUVA photochemotherapy is the method of choice. Also used at this stage are topical chemotherapy with nitrogen mustard in an ointment base (10 mg%) and total electron-beam therapy, singly or in combination. If isolated tumors should develop, these should be treated with local x-ray or electron beam therapy. For extensive plaque stage with multiple tumors, or in patients with lymphadenopathy or abnormal circulating T cells, electron-beam plus chemotherapy is probably the best combination, for now; randomized controlled studies of various combinations are now in progress. Also, extracorporeal PUVA photochemotherapy is being evaluated in patients with Sézary syndrome.

Table   TNM Classification of Mycosis Fungoides (MF) As Adopted for the U.S. National Cancer Institute Workshop on Cutaneous T-Cell Lymphomas (1979)

T: Skin	T0	Clinically and/or histologically suspicious lesions
	T1	Limited plaques, papules or eczematous patches covering less than 10% of the skin surface
	T2	Generalized plaques, papules or erythematous patches covering more than 10% of the skin surface
	T3	Tumors (one or more)
	T4	Generalized erythroderma
N: Lymph nodes	N0	No clinically abnormal peripheral nodes, pathology negative for MF
	N1	Clinically abnormal peripheral lymph nodes, pathology negative for MF
	N2	No clinically abnormal peripheral lymph nodes, pathology positive for MF
	N3	Clinically abnormal peripheral lymph nodes, pathology positive for MF
B: Blood	B0	Less than 5% atypical circulating lymphocytes
	B1	Greater than 5% atypical circulating lymphocytes
M: Visceral organs	M0	No visceral organ involvement
	M1	Histologically proven visceral involvement

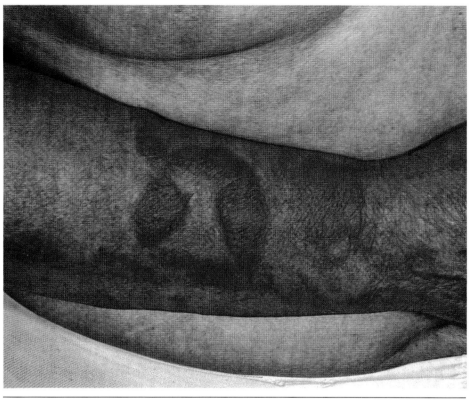

145 Mycosis fungoides

Physical examination: annular infiltration on the right arm of the same patient as shown in Figure 144

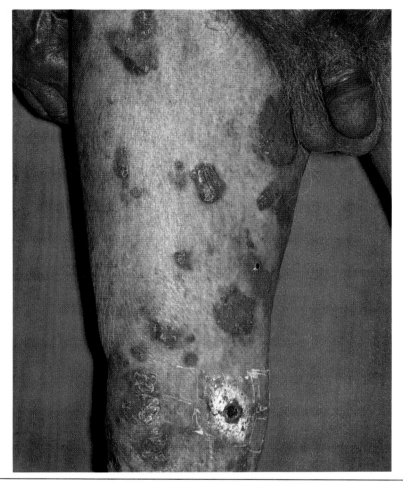

146 *Mycosis fungoides*

Patient Profile *Seventy-eight-year-old retired bricklayer*

History *The patient was originally treated for psoriasis, which gradually became atypical. Six years ago, a diagnosis of mycosis fungoides was established.*

Physical Examination *Disseminated over the upper leg, sharply but irregularly demarcated, infiltrated scaling plaques. One plaque is ulcerated in part.*

Differential Diagnosis *Psoriasis*

Histopathology *In the dermis, a bandlike lymphocytic infiltrate; several of the cells have a large, cerebriform nucleus. This infiltrate invades the epidermis.*

Clues *Clinical aspects, ulceration, histopathology*

Treatment and Course *Irradiation of the thicker infiltrated patches with soft x-rays; whole-body irradiation with ultrasoft x-rays; chemotherapy. Remained reasonably well for 5 years; died at age 84 from a cerebrovascular accident.*

Paget's Disease of the Nipple

This malignant neoplasm unilaterally involves the nipple, or areola, and simulates a chronic eczematous dermatitis.

EPIDEMIOLOGY

Age Thirty to fifty years
Sex Females, with rare examples in males

HISTORY

Duration of Lesions Insidious onset over several months or a year
Skin Symptoms Some itching or feeling of discomfort, complaints of soiling of the bra by the exudate

PHYSICAL EXAMINATION

Skin Lesions

TYPE Scaling plaque, rather sharply marginated, and when scale is removed, the surface is moist and oozing (see Figure 147)
COLOR Faintly red (see Figure 147)
PALPATION In early stages there is no induration, but, later, induration and infiltration develop and nodules may be palpated.
SHAPE Oval with irregular borders
DISTRIBUTION Single lesion localized to one nipple and areola. May uncommonly occur bilaterally

Miscellaneous Findings Regional lymph nodes are rarely found unless frank tumor (ulceration) is present in the epidermis. The breast tumor is an intraductal carcinoma.

DIFFERENTIAL DIAGNOSIS

Eczematous dermatitis of the nipples is usually bilateral and is without any induration and responds rapidly to topical corticosteroids. Nevertheless, be suspicious of Paget's disease if "eczema" persists for longer than 3 weeks.

DERMATOPATHOLOGY

Site Epidermis
Process Neoplastic. Typical large rounded cells with a large nucleus and without intercellular bridges (Paget's cells) which stain much lighter than surrounding keratinocytes.

TREATMENT

Mastectomy

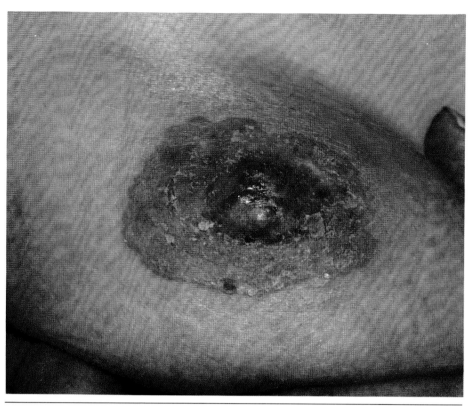

147 Paget's disease of the nipple

Patient Profile Forty-six-year-old female, three children

History For a year and a half, retraction of the right nipple and some discharge. Subsequently, eczematous changes. Treated by general physician with various ointments. No pain, no pruritus.

Physical Examination On the nipple and the areola mammae is a sharply demarcated erythematous area with slight scaling and an erosive and moist surface. There is a slight superficial induration. Axillary lymph nodes not palpable.

Differential Diagnosis Bowen's disease, superficial basal cell carcinoma, eczema

Laboratory and Special Examinations Biopsy: epidermis is somewhat thickened and covered by a thin keratotic layer; dispersed between the prickle cells are several PAS-positive and diastase-negative vacuolized Paget's cells, both single and in small clusters. With general examination and x-rays there were no signs of metastases.

Clues Long-standing, sharply demarcated eczema- or pyoderma-like lesion, not responding rapidly to topical treatment; typical histology

Treatment Mastectomy. Five years later the patient was still well.

XIX

Dermatologic

Artifacts

Dermatologic Artifacts (Factitial Dermatosis)

Dermatologic artifacts are lesions secretly produced by artificial means (fingernails, chemicals, cigarette butts) for gain, or as part of a severe psychiatric disturbance.

EPIDEMIOLOGY AND ETIOLOGY

Age Young adults
Sex More common in women
Occupation Nurses, medical students, pharmacists
Other Factors Severe mental disease such as senile dementia, schizophrenia, acute anxiety states (soldiers, etc.)

HISTORY

Duration of Lesions Weeks, months

PHYSICAL EXAMINATION

Skin and Hair

TYPE

Nodules (injected chemicals or bacteria)
Vesicles-bullae (chemicals)
Necrotic ulcers (chemicals, burns)
Alopecia (trichotillomania)

SHAPE Bizarre, "artificial" configurations, geometrical patterns (see Figure 148)
DISTRIBUTION Isolated single lesion or scattered discrete lesions
SITES OF PREDILECTION Arms, hands, face

DIFFERENTIAL DIAGNOSIS

The diagnosis of dermatologic artifacts is hazardous, and organic disease must be excluded by all possible means. Some disorders that appear as artifacts are *porphyria cutanea tarda, pemphigus, vasculitis, ulcers in lymphoma,* or *mycosis fungoides.*

MANAGEMENT

It is best to obtain a psychiatric consultation after all possibility of organic disease is excluded. There are serious malpractice implications.

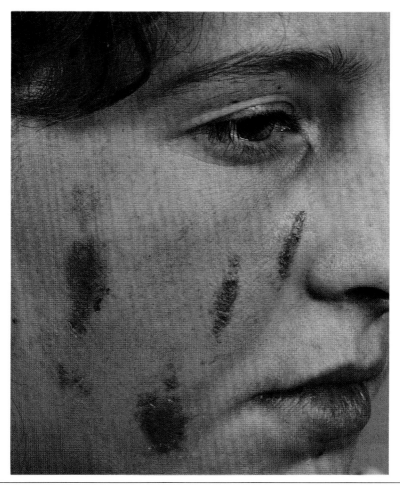

148 Neurotic excoriations

Patient Profile *Eighteen-year-old female working in a textile factory*

History *Since patient started her work in a textile factory 10 weeks ago, severe itching occurred on the face and also elsewhere.*

Physical Examination *On the face, irregularly disseminated, round and linear erosions*

Differential Diagnosis *Eczema*

Laboratory and Special Examinations *Bacterial cultures for erosions: sterile. Patch tests: negative.*

Psychologic Examination *Labile personality structure. After some time the patient confessed that she induces the lesions by rubbing.*

Clues *Clinical picture, compulsion to rub the face with a wet finger*

Prognosis *Varies with severity of emotional problem and other organic symptoms*

Appendices

PATHOGENESIS OF SKIN DISEASE

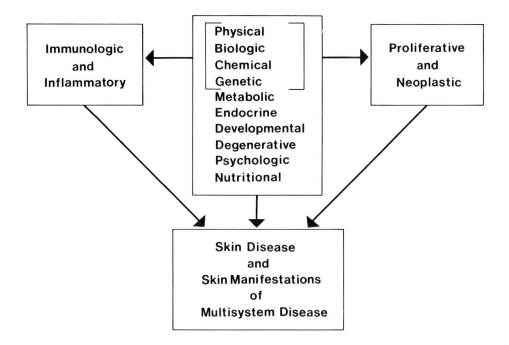

```
┌──────────────┐      ┌──────────────┐      ┌──────────────┐
│ Immunologic  │      │ Physical     │      │ Proliferative│
│    and       │ ◄─── │ Biologic     │ ───► │    and       │
│ Inflammatory │      │ Chemical     │      │ Neoplastic   │
└──────────────┘      │ Genetic      │      └──────────────┘
                      │ Metabolic    │
                      │ Endocrine    │
                      │ Developmental│
                      │ Degenerative │
                      │ Psychologic  │
                      │ Nutritional  │
                      └──────────────┘

              ┌──────────────────────┐
              │    Skin Disease      │
              │        and           │
              │ Skin Manifestations  │
              │         of           │
              │ Multisystem Disease  │
              └──────────────────────┘
```

Figure A-1 Listed above are the etiologic factors involved in dermatologic disorders. The interplay of these various etiologic factors is uniquely displayed in the skin. Some examples follow.

Psoriasis is a skin disorder of multiple etiologies. The etiologic factors include *genetic and metabolic,* in which there is a basic defect in the control of cell proliferation, with a marked increase in cell division leading to a massive production of white scales. At least one *biologic* agent, β-hemolytic streptococcus, causing pharyngitis, can induce an attack of acute generalized psoriasis. *Physical* (mechanical) trauma to the skin may provoke psoriatic lesions: This is known as an *isomorphic phenomenon* and characteristically occurs in psoriasis. Physical agents, such as ultraviolet radiation, can also bring about a marked flare of psoriasis. *Chemical* agents, such as practalone, can induce psoriasis, and *psychologic* factors, such as stress, may play a role.

In acne, no less than five of the etiologic factors listed in Figure A-1 interact to produce the disease. There is a basic *genetic* defect in the pilosebaceous apparatus, in which there is thought to be an alteration in the sensitivity of the sebaceous gland to androgens. There is a *biologic* etiology in the putative role of *Propionibacterium acnes* that multiplies in sebaceous glands. Furthermore, sebaceous glands are overactive because of *endocrine* stimulation (androgens). *Physical* factors—that is, pressure on the face with the hands or manipulation of the lesions—induce new lesions. *Psychologic* stress is believed by many experienced clinicians to be an important factor in the flare-up of quiescent acne, although this is difficult to prove. Finally, *chemical* agents, such as cutting oils and chlorinated hydrocarbons, can precipitate acne in susceptible persons.

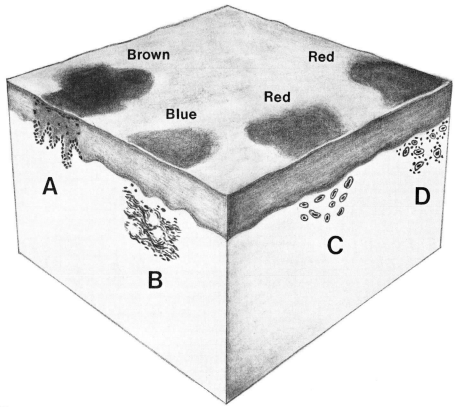

Macule

Figure B-1 A macule is a circumscribed area of change in normal skin color without elevation or depression of the surface relative to the surrounding skin. Macules may be of any size and are the result of (1) hypopigmentation (e.g., vitiligo) or hyperpigmentation—melanin (A) or hemosiderin (B)—such as café-au-lait spots and Mongolian spots (B), (2) permanent vascular abnormalities of the skin, as in a capillary hemangioma, or (3) transient capillary dilatation (erythema) (C). Pressure of a glass slide (diascopy) on the border of a red lesion is a simple and reliable method for detecting the extravasation of red blood cells. If the redness remains under pressure from the slide, the lesion may be purpuric (D); if the redness disappears, the lesion is erythematous and is due to vascular dilatation (C).

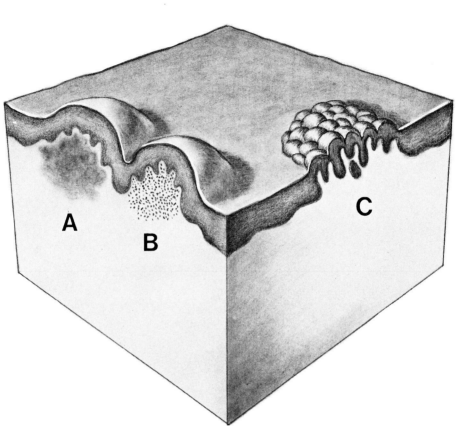

Papule

Figure B-2 A papule is a solid lesion, generally considered as less than 1 cm in diameter. Most of it is elevated above, rather than deep within, the plane of the surrounding skin. The elevation is caused by metabolic deposits (A) in the dermis, by localized infiltrates (B) in the dermis, or by localized hyperplasia of cellular elements (C) in the dermis or epidermis. Superficial papules with distinct borders are seen when the lesion is the result of an increase in the number of epidermal cells (C) or melanocytes. Deeper dermal papules resulting from cellular infiltrates have indistinct borders. The topography of a papule or plaque may consist of multiple, small, closely packed, or projected elevations that are known as a *vegetation* (C).

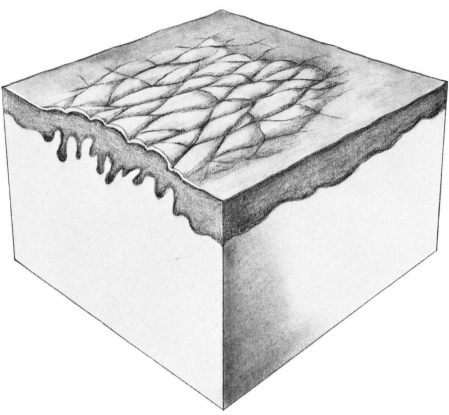

Plaque

Figure B-3 A plaque is an elevation above the skin surface that occupies a relatively large surface area in comparison with its height above the skin. Frequently it is formed by a confluence of papules as in psoriasis and mycosis fungoides. Lichenification is a proliferation of keratinocytes and stratum corneum forming a plaquelike structure. The skin appears thickened and the skin markings are accentuated. The process results from repeated rubbing of the skin and frequently develops in persons with atopy. Lichenification occurs typically in eczematous dermatitis but is also found in psoriasis and mycosis fungoides.

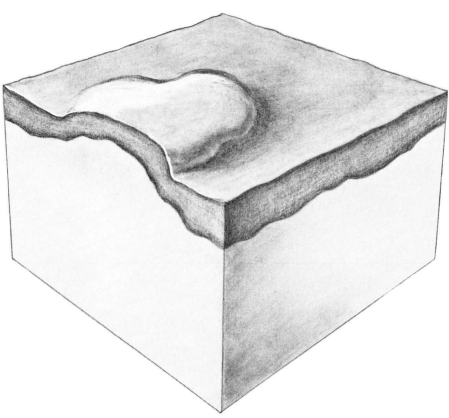

Wheal

Figure B-4 A wheal is a rounded or flat-topped, pale-red elevation in the skin that is characteristically evanescent, disappearing within hours. Wheals that persist longer than 24 hr should be examined histologically for the presence of necrotizing angiitis. Observation of the borders of wheals that have been traced with a skin-marking pencil reveals that the wheals shift relatively rapidly from the involved to the uninvolved adjacent areas. Wheals are the result of edema in the upper layer of the dermis.

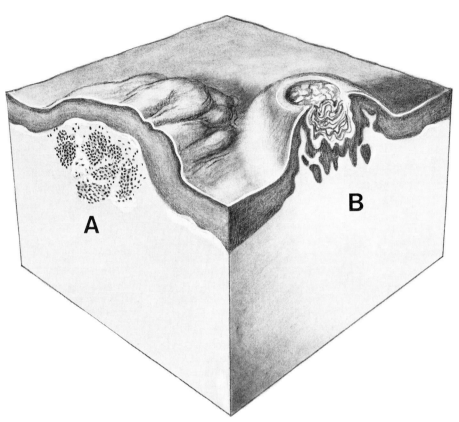

Nodule

Figure B-5 A nodule is a palpable, solid, round, or ellipsoidal lesion deeper than a papule and is in the dermis or subcutaneous tissue (A) or in the epidermis (B). The depth of involvement and the palpability rather than the diameter differentiates a nodule from a papule. Nodules result from infiltrates (A), neoplasms (B), or metabolic deposits in the dermis or subcutaneous tissue and often indicate systemic disease. Tuberculosis, the deep mycoses, lymphoma, and metastatic neoplasms, for example, can present as cutaneous nodules. Therefore, a biopsy should be performed on unidentified persistent nodules, and a portion of excised tissue should be ground in a sterile mortar and cultured for fungi and bacteria. Nodules can develop as a result of a benign or malignant proliferation of keratinocytes, as in keratoacanthoma (B), verruca vulgaris, and squamous cell and basal cell carcinoma.

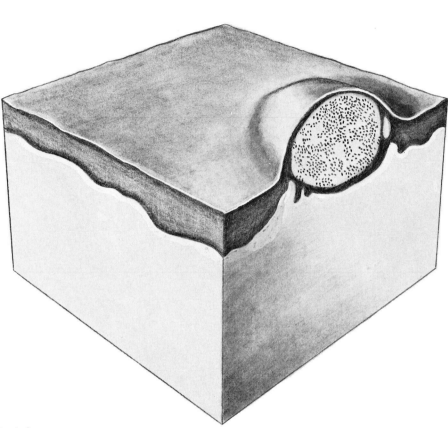

Pustule

Figure B-6 A pustule is a circumscribed elevation of the skin that contains a purulent exudate that may be white, yellow, or greenish yellow. This process may arise in a hair follicle or independently. Pustules may vary in size and shape; follicular pustules, however, are always conical and usually contain a hair in the center. The vesicular lesions of the viral diseases (varicella, variola, vaccinia, herpes simplex, and herpes zoster) may secondarily become pustular. A Gram stain and culture should be done on all pustules.

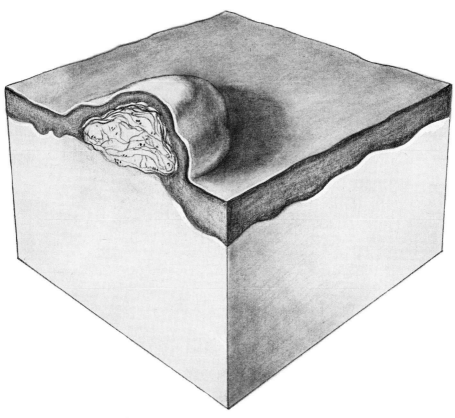

Vesicle (Subepidermal)

Figure B-7 A vesicle (less than 0.5 cm) or a bulla (more than 0.5 cm) is a circumscribed elevated lesion containing fluid. Often the walls are so thin that they are translucent, and the serum, lymph fluid, blood, or extracellular fluid can be seen. Vesicles and bullae arise from a cleavage at various levels of the skin; the cleavage may be within the epidermis (i.e., intraepidermal vesication), or at the epidermal-dermal interface (i.e., subepidermal), as in this figure.

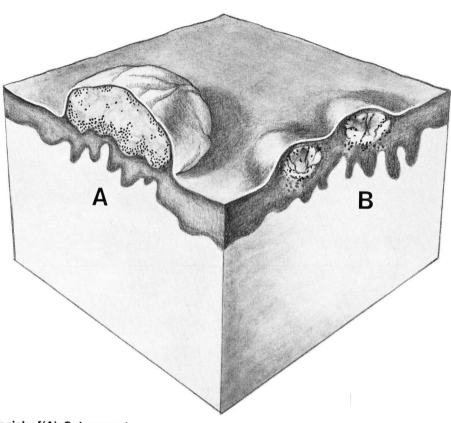

Vesicle [(A) Subcorneal, (B) Spongiotic]

Figure B-8 When the cleavage is just beneath the stratum corneum, a subcorneal vesicle or bulla results (A), as in impetigo and subcorneal pustular dermatosis. Intraepidermal vesication may result from intercellular edema, or spongiosis (B), as characteristically seen in delayed-hypersensitivity reactions of the epidermis (e.g., in contact eczematous dermatitis) and in dyshidrotic eczema (B). Spongiotic vesicles may or may not be observed clinically as vesicles.

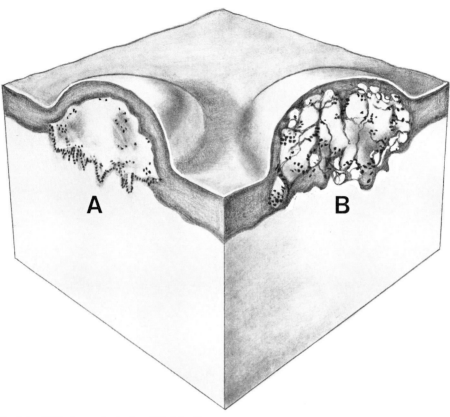

Vesicle [(A) Acantholytic, (B) Viral]

Figure B-9 Loss of intercellular bridges, or desmosomes, is known as *acantholysis* (A), and this type of intraepidermal vesication is seen in the vesicles or bullae of pemphigus vulgaris; the cleavage is usually just above the basal layer, as in pemphigus vulgaris, but may occur just below the subcorneal layer, as in pemphigus foliaceus. Viruses cause a curious "ballooning degeneration" of epidermal cells (B), as in herpes zoster, herpes simplex, variola, and varicella. Viral bullae often have a depressed ("umbilicated") center.

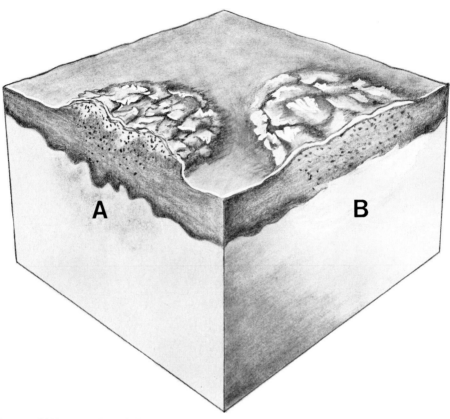

Crusts [(A) Impetigo, (B) Ecthyma]

Figure B-10 Crusts result when serum or blood or purulent exudate dries on the skin surface. Crusts may be thin, delicate, and friable (A) or thick and adherent (B). Crusts are yellow when formed from dried serum, green or yellow-green when formed from purulent exudate, or brown or dark red when formed from blood. Superficial crusts occur as honey-colored, delicate, glistening particulates on the surface (A) and are typically found in impetigo. When the exudate involves the entire epidermis, the crusts may be thick and adherent, and this condition is known as *ecthyma* (B).

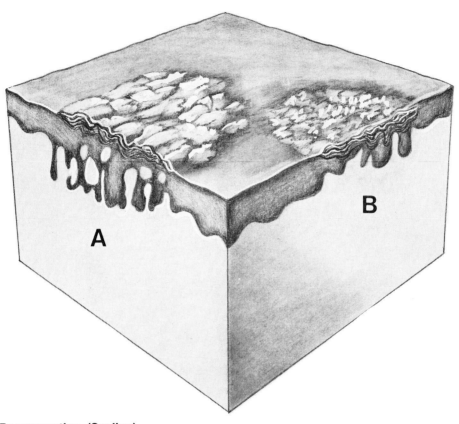

Desquamation (Scaling)
[(A) Psoriasis, (B) Solar Keratosis]

Figure B-11 Epidermal cells are completely replaced every 27 days. The end product of this holocrine process is the stratum corneum. This outermost layer of skin, the stratum corneum, normally does not contain nuclei and is imperceptibly lost. With an increased rate of proliferation of epidermal cells, as in psoriasis, the stratum corneum is not formed normally and the outermost layers of the skin retain the nuclei (parakeratosis). These desquamating layers of skin are seen clinically as scales (A). Densely adherent scales that have a gritty feel (like sandpaper) result from a localized increase in the stratum corneum and are a characteristic of solar keratosis (B).

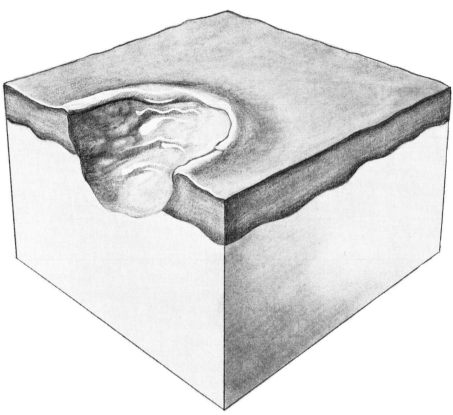

Ulcer

Figure B-12 An ulcer is a lesion in which there has been destruction of the epidermis and the upper papillary layer of the dermis. Certain features that are helpful in determining the cause of ulcers include location, borders, base, discharge, and any associated topographic features of the lesions, such as nodules, excoriations, varicosities, hair distribution, presence or absence of sweating, and pulses.

Appendix C: Special Clinical and Laboratory Aids to Dermatologic Diagnosis

AIDS IN SKIN AND HAIR CLINICAL EXAMINATION

1. *Magnification with hand lens* To examine lesions for fine morphologic detail, it is necessary to use a magnifier (2 to 7X) or a binocular microscope (5 to 40X). Magnification is especially effective in the diagnosis of lupus erythematosus (follicular plugging), lichen planus (Wickham's striae), carcinomas, and malignant melanoma.

2. *Oblique lighting* of the skin lesion, done in a darkened room, is often required to detect slight degrees of elevation or depression, and it is useful in the visualization of the surface configuration of lesions and in estimating the extent of the eruption.

3. *Subdued lighting* in the examining room enhances the contrast between circumscribed hypopigmented or hyperpigmented lesions and normal skin.

4. *Wood's lamp* (ultraviolet long-wave light, "black" light) is valuable in the diagnosis of certain skin and hair diseases and of porphyria. Long-wave ultraviolet radiation can be obtained by fitting a high-pressure mercury lamp with a specially compounded filter made of nickel oxide and silica (Wood's filter); this filter is very opaque to all light except for a band between 320 and 400 nm. The lamp with this filter produces adequate long-wave ultraviolet radiation. When the ultraviolet waves emitted by Wood's lamp (360 nm) impinge on the skin, a visible fluorescence occurs. Wood's lamp is particularly useful in the detection of the fluorescence of dermatophytosis in the hair shaft. A presumptive diagnosis of porphyria can be made if a pinkish-red or orange-red fluorescence is demonstrated in urine examined with Wood's lamp; addition of dilute hydrochloric acid greatly intensifies the fluorescence. Wood's lamp also helps to estimate the variation in the lightness of lesions in relation to the normal skin color, in both dark-skinned and fair-skinned peoples; e.g., the lesions seen in tuberous sclerosis and tinea versicolor are hypomelanotic and are not as light as the lesions seen in vitiligo, which are amelanotic. Circumscribed hypermelanosis, such as a freckle and melasma, is much more evident under Wood's lamp. On the other hand, dermal melanin as in a Mongolian sacral spot does not become accentuated under Wood's lamp. Therefore it is possible to localize the site of melanin by use of the Wood's lamp.

5. *Diascopy* consists of firmly pressing a microscope slide or a piece of clear plastic over a skin lesion. The examiner will find this procedure of special value in determining whether the red color of a macule or papule is due to capillary dilatation (erythema) or to extravasation of blood (purpura). Diascopy is also useful for the detection of the glassy yellow-brown appearance of papules in sarcoidosis, tuberculosis of the skin, lymphoma, and granuloma annulare.

6. *Acetowhitening* facilitates detection of subclinical penile warts. Ninety to 100 percent of male partners of HPV-infected females with genital warts are also infected. Gauze saturated with 5% acetic acid (white vinegar) is wrapped around the penis. After 5 to 10 minutes the penis is inspected with a colposcope or 10 × hand lens. Warts appear as small white papules.

CLINICAL TESTS

1. *Darier's sign* is "positive" when a brown macular or the most slightly papular lesion of urticaria pigmentosa (mastocytosis) becomes a palpable wheal after being rubbed with the blunt end of an instrument such as a pen. The wheal may not appear for 5 to 10 min.

2. *Patch testing* is used to document and validate a diagnosis of allergic contact sensitization and identify the causative agent. It may also be of value as a screening procedure in some patients with chronic or bizarre eczematous eruptions (e.g., hand and foot dermatoses). It is a unique means of in vivo reproduction of disease in diminutive proportions, for sensitization affects the whole body and may therefore be elicited at any cutaneous site. The patch test is easier and safer than a "use test" with a questionable allergen, for test items can be applied in low concentrations in small areas of skin for short periods of time. See textbooks on contact dermatitis.

MICROSCOPE EXAMINATION OF SCALES, CRUSTS, SERUM, AND HAIR

1. *Gram's stains and cultures of exudates* should be made in lesions suspected of being bacterial or yeast (*Can-*

dida albicans) infections. Ulcers and nodules require a scalpel biopsy in which a wedge of tissue consisting of all three layers of skin is obtained; the biopsy specimen is minced in a sterile mortar and the tissue is then cultured for bacteria (including typical and atypical mycobacteria) and fungi.

2. *Microscope examination* for mycelia should be made of the roofs of vesicles or of the scales (the advancing borders are preferable) or of the hair. The tissue is cleared with 10% potassium hydroxide and warmed gently (see Figure 74 for illustration of mycelia). Fungal cultures on Sabouraud's medium should be made.

3. *Microscope examination of cells obtained from the base of vesicles* (Tzanck test) may reveal the presence of giant epithelial cells and multinucleated giant cells (containing 10 to 12 nuclei) in herpes simplex, herpes zoster, and varicella. Material from the base of a vesicle obtained by gentle curettage with a scalpel is smeared on a glass slide, stained with Giemsa's or Wright's stain, and examined to determine whether there are giant epithelial cells, which are diagnostic.

4. *Laboratory diagnosis of scabies* The diagnosis of scabies is usually immediately considered in a patient with intractable generalized pruritus and with papules and excoriations distributed in characteristic locations, on the flexor aspects of the wrists and on the buttocks and genitalia; the diagnosis is established by identification of the mite, or ova or feces, in skin scrapings removed from the papules or burrows (see Figure 105). The burrow, a unique lesion, is a linear or serpiginous elevation of skin in the form of a ridge, 0.5 to 1.0 cm in length. These occur on the anterior surface of the wrist, in the webs of the fingers, or on the ulnar border of the hands. If burrows are not present, select a papule. The mineral oil technique is excellent for isolating the mite. Using a sterile scalpel blade on which a drop of sterile mineral oil has been placed, apply oil to the surface of the burrow or papule. Scrape the papule or burrow vigorously (about six times) in order to remove the entire top of the papule. Tiny flecks of blood will appear in the oil. Transfer the oil to a coverglass and examine for mites, ova, and feces. The mites are 0.2 to 0.4 mm in size and have four pairs of legs (see Figure 105).

5. *Dark-field examination of serum from ulcers* on the male or female genitalia (es-pecially the penis, anus, vulva, and cervix) is essential for detection of *Treponema pallidum*. Dark-field examinations are not worthwhile in material obtained from the oral cavity because of the presence of nonpathogenic treponemas indistinguishable from *T. pallidum.* (A serologic test for syphilis is mandatory for all patients with generalized erythematous and scaling eruptions, including all patients with the diagnosis of pityriasis rosea.)

BIOPSY OF THE SKIN

Biopsy of the skin is one of the simplest, most rewarding diagnostic techniques in medical practice because of the easy accessibility of the skin and the variety of techniques for study of the excised specimen (e.g., immunofluorescence, electron microscopy).

The selection of the site of the biopsy is based primarily on the stage of the eruption, and early lesions are usually more typical; this is especially important in vesiculobullous eruptions (e.g., pemphigus, herpes simplex) in which the lesion should be no more than 24 hr old. However, older lesions (2 to 6 weeks) are often more characteristic in discoid lupus erythematosus.

A common technique for diagnostic biopsy is the use of a 4.0-mm punch, a small tubular knife much like a corkscrew, which by rotating movements between the thumb and index finger cuts through the epidermis, dermis, and subcutaneous tissue; the base is cut off with scissors. If immunofluorescence is indicated (as, for example, in bullous diseases or lupus erythematosus), a special technique is necessary and the laboratory should be consulted.

For nodules, however, a surgeon should remove a large wedge by excision including subcutaneous tissue. Furthermore, all nodules, regardless of size, should be bisected, one half for histology, the other half sent in a sterile container for bacterial and mycotic cultures using a tissue mince.

Specimens for light microscopy should be fixed immediately in buffered neutral formalin. A brief but detailed summary of the clinical history and lesions should accompany the specimen. Biopsy is indicated in all skin lesions that are suspected of being neoplasms, in all bullous disorders using immunofluorescence simultaneously, and in all dermatologic disorders in which a specific diagnosis is not possible by clinical examination alone.

Appendix D: Skin Phototypes (SPT)

A careful history of the reaction of each patient to sun exposure—tendency to sunburn and capacity to tan—enables the physician to categorize Caucasians with white skin by *Skin Phototypes (SPT)* and thereby to be able to estimate the relative risk of the development of their acute and chronic changes related to ultraviolet radiation exposure, including melanoma and nonmelanoma skin cancer.

There is a special high-risk normal white-skinned population who have poor tolerance to sunlight (SPT I). These are most often light-skinned people with red or blond hair, blue eyes, and freckles (ephelides). Identification of this subgroup who are genetically inadequately protected from sunlight signals a group of people who must use protective measures. Heavily tanned, swarthy-skinned (SPT IV) people have little or no sunburn response to sun exposure except to develop an "immediate" tan; often these people have only occasional and limited need for ancillary sun protection.

How do we identify the white population at high risk for the development of sun-induced skin changes, including skin cancer? A simple working classification has been proposed (Table D-1) that is based, not on the phenotype (i.e., hair and eye color), but on how patients describe responses to an *initial* sun exposure—three minimum erythema doses (MED) of about 1 hr in northern latitudes in the summer between the hours of 1100 and 1400. If we ask two questions about their responses to three MED exposures— (1) "How much painful sunburn do you have after 24 hours?"; (2) "How much tan will you develop in a week?"—there are two groups of the white population with a clear-cut answer. One group will reply "a painful burn at 24 hours and no tan at seven days." This is SPT I; they may have dark hair and brown eyes! Another group will respond "no burn at 24 hours and a good tan at seven days." This group is called SPT IV. A subgroup of SPT I will answer "a painful burn at 24 hours (the same as SPT I response) and possibly a light tan at seven days"; this group is SPT II. A subgroup of SPT IV will testify to "a slightly tender burn at 24 hours and a good tan at seven days"; this is SPT III and is the largest group. SPT I and II are at high risk for sun-induced skin damage; SPT IV persons have a low risk for sun-induced skin damage; SPT III persons are at moderate risk, but persons in this group often have a history of repeated and prolonged sun exposure— often to deliberately obtain a cosmetic tan!

Repeated solar insults can ultimately result in skin cancer and, in addition, to a syndrome we have called *dermatoheliosis*, especially in SPT I and SPT II persons. Dermatoheliosis describes the effects of repeated exposures to the sun on normal skin.

Table D-1 Classification of Sun-Reactive Skin Phototypes in Persons with White Skin

Skin Phototype*	Erythema and tanning reactions[†] to first exposure in summer to 3 minimum erythema doses (MED) (MED = 15-30 min of noon summer sun)
I	Always burn, never tan
II	Usually burn, tan less than average (with difficulty)
III	Sometimes mild burn, tan about average
IV	Rarely burn, tan more than average (with ease)

*SPT I and SPT II persons all have pale skin color and often but not always have blue eyes, red scalp hair, and may or may not have freckling; however, some persons with dark brown hair and blue or green eyes have SPT I and SPT II sun reactions.

[†]At ages 12 to 40 years.

Sources   Fitzpatrick TB: Soleil et peau. *Journal de Médecine Esthétique* 2(7):33–34 (1975)

Fitzpatrick TB: The validity and practicality of sun-reactive Skin Types I–VI. *Arch Dermatol* 124:869–871, 1988

These effects occur following the first exposures in early life and are cumulative and irreversible. The magnitude and variety of the effects depend on the natural defense mechanisms and on whether or not susceptible persons use effective topical sun-protective agents throughout life. The dermatoheliosis syndrome is a polymorphic response to sun exposure of various components of the skin: (1) the *vascular system* of the dermis, with acute, transient, mediator-induced vasodilatation (sunburn erythema) or permanent dilatation of vessels (telangiectasia); (2) the *keratinocytes* of the epidermis, leading to localized atypical keratinocytic hyperplasia (solar keratosis); (3) the *melanocytes* of the epidermis, leading to macular pigmented lesions with sharply irregular borders and variegated brown color (freckles) and to isolated smooth-bordered, uniformly brown macules (solar lentigo); and (4) the *connective tissue components* of the dermis, collagen, and elastic tissue, leading to wrinkling, roughening, and yellowing of the skin.

Dermatoheliosis, which is analogous to pneumoconiosis, is a preventable environmental hazard that can potentially affect the health of approximately 25 percent (SPT I and SPT II) of the population of the United States. Excessive exposure to the skin in normal white persons leads to acute and chronic dermatoheliosis. Persons at risk need to be identified at an early age and need to be made aware of the noxious long-term effects of the sun: (1) avoiding exposure during the peak flux of UVB in the middle hours of the day, and (2) using substantive and effective topical sunscreens (SPF 15) in a daily program of self-protection.

Appendix E: Dermatomes

Figure E-1 The cutaneous fields of peripheral nerves. (*a*) The segmental innervation of the skin from the anterior aspect. The uppermost dermatome adjoins the cutaneous field of the mandibular division of the trigeminal nerve. The arrows indicate the lateral extensions of dermatome 13. (*b*) The dermatomes from the posterior view. Note the absence of cutaneous innervation by the first cervical segment. Arrows in the axillary regions indicate the lateral extent of dermatome T3; those in the region of the vertebral column point to the first thoracic, the first lumbar, and the first sacral spinous processes. (*After Foerster in Haymaker W, Woodhall B: Peripheral Nerve Injuries, 2d ed. Saunders, Philadelphia/London, 1953.*)

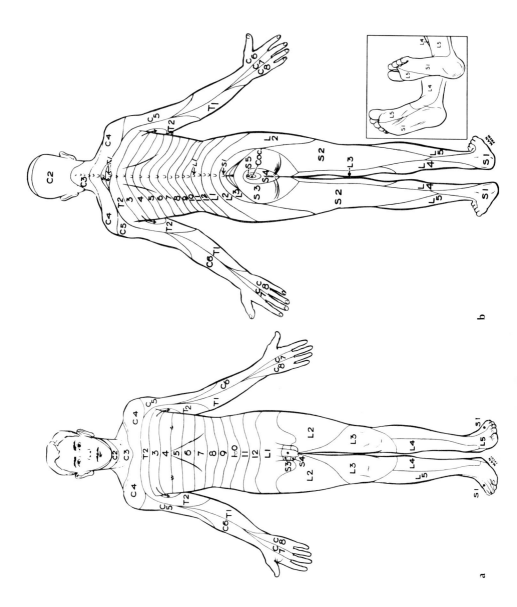

Appendix F: Malignant Melanoma

RECOMMENDATIONS FOR THE MANAGEMENT OF PIGMENTED LESIONS TO FACILITATE EARLY DIAGNOSIS OF MALIGNANT MELANOMA[1]

For the Examining Physician

A. Histologic diagnosis is necessary in all pigmented lesions with the following three physical characteristics–the hallmarks of malignancy in a pigmented lesion:

1. Irregularity of the borders: with pseudopods, a notch, or even a "maple leaf" configuration (see Figures 139 and 140)
2. An irregular array of colors: a gradation of red, gray, or blue, admixed with brown or black, displayed in a disorderly, haphazard pigment pattern. *Exceptions:* black nodules with uniform borders, irregularly pigmented lesions with uniform borders
3. Increases in size.

B. All congenital melanocytic nevi should be considered for excision, regardless of size. Larger lesions should be followed with photography until they can be excised some time before puberty. The timing of excision for small congenital lesions will depend on the clinical characteristics (light brown, uniform color is a sign of benignancy), whether general anesthesia is needed, and on the disability that will result from surgery. All giant nevi should be removed whenever possible.

C. Excision of all acquired nevocytic nevi that cannot be easily observed: anogenital area, mucous membranes (nose, mouth, vagina), and scalp. All pigmented lesions, raised or flat!

D. Any pigmented lesion striking a physician's eye as "out of the ordinary" should be further evaluated (i.e., excision or referral for same).

E. All patients with a history of melanoma should be thoroughly examined for atypical melanocytic nevi (dysplastic nevi) and for the appearance of new primary melanomas. Patients with dysplastic nevi should be followed at 12-month intervals.

F. All blood relatives of patients with melanoma should be examined for dysplastic nevi and early primary melanoma. (The presence of a family history increases the risk 12-fold for an individual.)

G. All white patients presenting for any problem should be examined for the presence of large melanocytic nevi (greater than 1.0 cm), for dysplastic nevi, and for nevi on the scalp, mucous membrane, and anogenital area. All black persons should be examined for dysplastic lesions of the soles, nail beds, and mucous membranes.

Advice to the Patient

The following advice to all persons should be made regarding pigmented lesions.

Seek immediate examination for the following.

Any raised (palpable) pigmented "mole" present at birth

Any newly arising pigmented lesion after age 30

Any changing lesion—in size, color, or border

Any mole that itches or is tender

All moles that are difficult to observe: scalp, mucous membranes (nose, mouth, vagina), anogenital area

Any pigmented lesion considered as "ugly" because of its size, color pattern, or borders

A family history of melanoma

Skin Phototype I or II

Skin Phototype I and II persons should *never* sunbathe. Persons with dysplastic nevi should *never* sunbathe, regardless of skin type. Sunscreens with a sun protective factor (SPF) of 15 should be used in all persons with Skin Phototype I and II and in all patients with dysplastic nevi or with a previous history of melanoma.

---

[1] Melanoma Cooperative Group (Harvard).

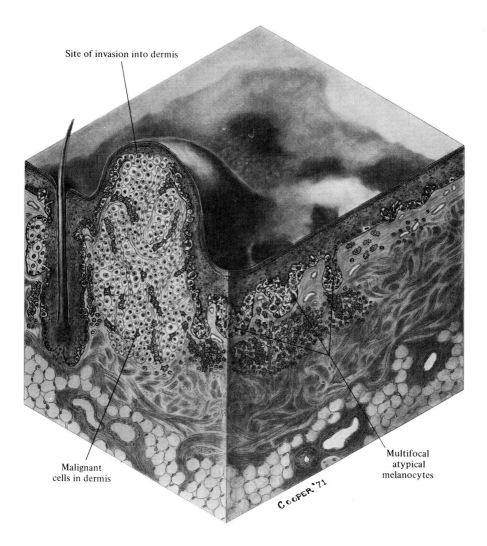

Site of invasion into dermis

Malignant cells in dermis

Multifocal atypical melanocytes

COOPER '71

PRIMARY MELANOMA OF THE SKIN: THREE MAJOR TYPES

Figure F-1 Lentigo maligna melanoma. Illustrated is a large, flat, variegated, freckle-like *macule* (not elevated above the plane of the skin) with irregular borders. The tan areas show increased numbers of melanocytes, usually atypical and bizarre and distributed along the basal layer; at certain places in the dermis, malignant melanocytes have invaded and formed huge nests. At the left is a large nodule which is comprised of large epithelioid cells in this illustration; the nodules of all three types of melanoma are indistinguishable from each other.

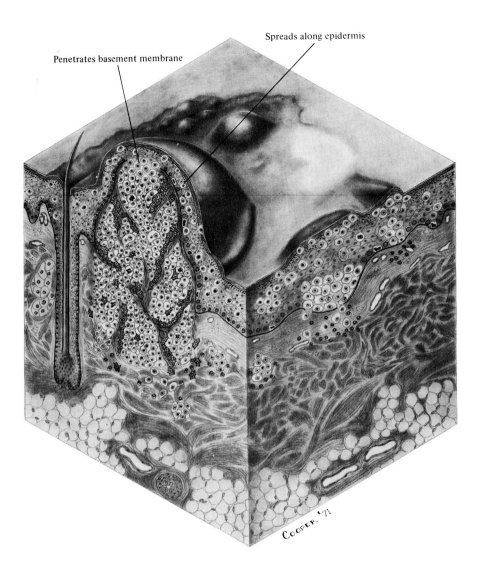

Penetrates basement membrane

Spreads along epidermis

COOPER '71

Figure F-2 Superficial spreading melanoma. The border is irregular and elevated throughout its entirety; biopsy of the area surrounding the large nodule shows a pagetoid distribution of large melanocytes throughout the dermis, occurring singly or in nests, and uniformly atypical. On the left is a large nodule, and scattered throughout the surrounding portion of the nodule are smaller papular and nodular areas. The nodule on the left shows malignant melanocytes that are very large, have an abundance of cytoplasm, and often have regularly dispersed fine particles of melanin. The nodules may also show spindle cells or small malignant melanocytes as in lentigo maligna melanoma and nodular melanoma.

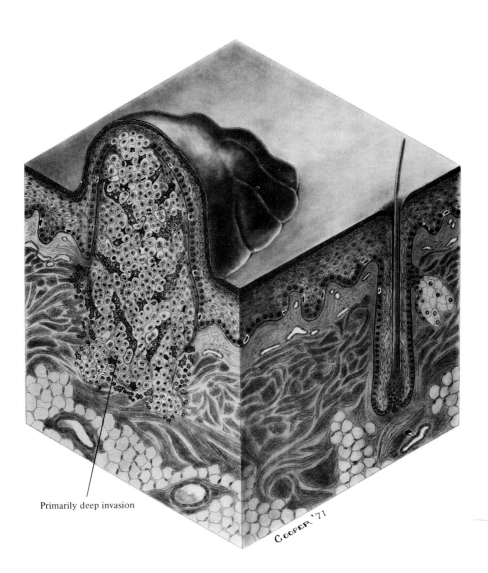

Primarily deep invasion

COOPER '71

Figure F-3 Nodular melanoma. This arises at the dermal-epidermal junction and extends laterally in the dermis; intraepidermal growth is present only in a small group of tumor cells that conjointly are also invading the underlying dermis. The epidermis lateral to the areas of this invasion does not demonstrate atypical melanocytes. As in lentigo maligna melanoma and superficial spreading melanoma, the tumor may show large epithelioid cells, spindle cells, small malignant melanocytes, or mixtures of all three.

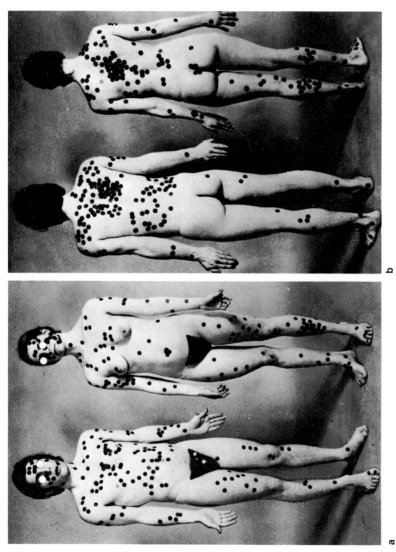

Figure F-4 Localization of malignant melanoma in 731 males and females.

SUMMARY DATA ON MALIGNANT MELANOMA OF SKIN

I. **INCIDENCE:** Two percent of all cancers (excluding nonmelanoma skin cancer)
- A. Overall annual crude incidence rates (United States)
  1. Caucasians   9 per 100,000 population per year
  2. Blacks   0.6 per 100,000 population per year
- B. Increasing with time (Connecticut Registry)
  1. 1935–1939   1.2 per 100,000 population per year
  2. 1965–1969   4.8 per 100,000 population per year
  3. 1976–1977   7.2 per 100,000 population per year
  4. 1980–1981   9.0 per 100,000 population per year
- C. Latitude-dependent crude incidence rates
  1. Northern United States (Connecticut)   9 per 100,000 population per year
  2. Southern United States (Arizona)   26 per 100,000 population per year

II. **FREQUENCY FOR TYPE OF MELANOMA**
- A. Superficial spreading   70 percent
- B. Nodular   16 percent
- C. Lentigo maligna melanoma   5 percent
- D. Unclassified (includes acral lentiginous type)   10 percent

III. **MORTALITY:** Overall deaths (United States 6000); melanoma represents 1 to 2 percent of all cancer deaths

GUIDELINES FOR BIOPSY, SURGICAL TREATMENT, AND FOLLOW-UP OF PATIENTS WITH MELANOMA

I. **BIOPSY**
- A. Total excisional biopsy with narrow margins—optimal biopsy procedure, where possible
- B. Incisional or punch acceptable when total excisional biopsy cannot be performed or when lesion is large, requiring extensive surgery to remove the entire lesion

II. **LENTIGO MALIGNA MELANOMA—ALL LEVELS**
1. Excise with a 1-cm or greater margin beyond the clinically visible lesion or biopsy scar provided the flat component does not involve a major organ (e.g., the eye), in which lesser margins are acceptable.
2. Excise down to or including the fascia or to the underlying muscle where fascia is absent. Skin flaps or skin grafts may be used for closure. Margin width greater than 1 cm is determined by location; a greater margin should be obtained if technically possible.
3. No node dissection recommended unless nodes are clinically palpable and tumor-bearing.

III. **SUPERFICIAL SPREADING MELANOMA, NODULAR MELANOMA, AND ACRAL MELANOMA**
- A. Thickness less than 0.85 mm, no clinical or histopathologic evidence of regression:
  1. Excise or reexcise the lesion with at least a 1.5-cm margin from the lesion edge.
  2. Excise down to or including the fascia or to the underlying muscle where fascia is absent. Graft will usually not be necessary.
  3. No node dissection is recommended unless nodes are clinically suspicious for tumor.
- B. Thickness more than 0.85 mm:
  1. Excise or reexcise the lesion with a 3.0-cm margin from the lesion edge, except on the face.
  2. Excise down to or including the fascia or to the underlying muscle where fascia is absent. Graft is usually required.
  3. Elective nodal dissection is optional, at the descretion of the surgeon. Regional lymph node dissections are done in some centers for melanomas with a thickness of >1.7 mm.

IV. Follow-up
1. Every 3 months for 2 years, with chest x-ray once yearly
2. Every 6 months for the third through the fifth years
3. Annually thereafter

Table F-1 Prognosis and Frequency of Follow-Up of Clinical Stage I* Melanoma

Thickness Group (mm)	Five-Year Cumulative Survival, %	Ten-Year Cumulative Survival, %	Follow-Up Frequency (months)	Follow-Up Duration (years)
0.01–0.75	99	97.8	6	2
0.76–1.50	95	90.7	6	5
1.51–3.00	84	81.6	3	5
≥ 3.01	70	47.2	3	5
> 4.0	44	N.A.	2–3	5
Overall	86.4	81.5	Annual follow-up for life	

*Localized disease without palpable regional lymph nodes.
Note: For lesions of thickness >1.7, a CAT scan should be done and regional node dissection is recommended

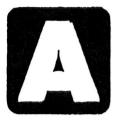

ASYMMETRY in shape—one half unlike the other

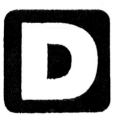

BORDER is irregular—edges irregularly scalloped

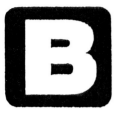

COLOR is mottled—haphazard display of colors: shades of brown, black, gray, and white

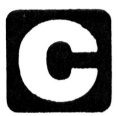

DIAMETER is usually large—greater than the tip of a pencil eraser (6.0 mm)

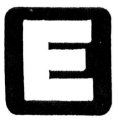

ELEVATION is almost always present—surface distortion, subtle or obvious, assessed by side-lighting. Acral lentiginous lesions may be flat.

Appendix H: Risk Factors of White Adults for Cutaneous Melanoma*

Mortality rates of primary melanoma in white persons for single years from 1975 to 1982 are rising at the rate of 3% per year in males. In males living in Connecticut, ages 30 to 49, primary melanoma is the second most prevalent of all cancers—the first being cancer of the testis. Physicians and health care providers are in a unique position to improve the survival rates of melanoma of the skin because not only are the characteristics of early melanoma well delineated (see page 393) and easily detected, but there are now known the characteristics of the population at risk. The following factors list the degree of risk for persons with the risk factor compared with persons without the risk factor. (With a relative risk of 1.0, there is no increased risk.)

	Risk
1. **Changing "mole"**	Very high

This is seen as a change in color—especially darkening and mottling, in a previously uniformly colored mole. Also, an increase in size (height or diameter) and change in borders (becoming irregular); these are early signs of a mole changing to a melanoma.

2. **Large, irregularly shaped, pigmented lesions**
   A. Clark's dysplastic melanocytic nevi (see page 292):

With a history of melanoma in the family	148 ×
Without a history of melanoma in the family	27 ×
B. Lentigo maligna (see page 342)	10 ×

3. **Congenital mole** (see page 296) — 21 ×
Lesions >1.5 cm are either dysplastic melanocytic nevi or congenital melanocytic nevi

4. **Family history of melanoma of the skin in parents, siblings, or children** — 8 ×

5. **Inability to tan normally** — 3 ×
Skin Phototypes I and II (see page 383). There also appears to be increased risk of persons with a history of excessive sun exposure, especially obtained during childhood.

---

*Adapted in part from Rhodes AR et al: Risk factors for cutaneous melanoma. JAMA 258:3146–3154, 1987.

Appendix I: Daily Doses of Antibiotics

Table G-1 Daily Doses of Antibiotics

	Pediatric		Adult	
Antibiotic	Oral (in 4 doses)	IM	Oral (in 4 doses)	IM
Cephalexin	25–50 mg/kg		1–4 g	
Erythromycin*	30–50 mg/kg		2–4 g	
Lincomycin*	30–60 mg/kg	10–20 mg/kg in 1–2 doses	1.2–2.4 g	2.4 g in 2–4 doses
Penicillin V-K†	25,000–50,000 units/kg		3–4 g	
Penicillin G	0.5–2 million units/kg (½–1 h *before* meals)	20,000–50,000 units/kg		2–4 million units
Benzathine penicillin		600,000–1.2 million units, single injection	600,000–1.2 million units, single injection	
Procaine penicillin		100,000 units/kg in 2–4 doses		
Oxacillin†	50–100 mg/kg	50–100 mg/kg in 2–3 doses	4–6 g	
Cloxacillin	50–100 mg/kg		4–6 g	
Dicloxacillin†	12.5–25 mg/kg		2–3 g	
Nafcillin	25–50 mg/kg	50 mg/kg in 2 doses	4 g	
Tetracycline HCl	20–50 mg/kg		2 g	
Minocycline‡	—	—	50–100 mg bid	

*For allergic patient.
†Preferred.
‡Not for children younger than 10 years.

Index of
Differential Diagnosis
by Regions

NOTE: Anatomic, physiologic, and biochemical factors indigenous to certain areas may account for the localization of skin diseases on the face, perianal area, ear, and other areas. Since a considerable number of skin diseases may be limited to specific regions, the following differential lists of diseases classified by site should prove helpful in narrowing the number of possible diagnoses. The diseases listed below are ones discussed in this book; it is not a complete differential diagnosis of the various body regions.

See also the Subject Index, which follows the Topographical Index.

INGUINAL REGIONS *(Cont.)*

Erosions
Moniliasis, 214, 216, 217, 223
Pemphigus vulgaris, 106–109
Impetigo, 174, 175

Lichenification
Chronic eczematous dermatitis, 6, 7, 371

PUBIC AREA

Macules
Seborrheic dermatitis (scaling), 66–73

Papules or Plaques
Lichen simplex chronicus, 22, 23
Psoriasis, 46–48
Seborrheic dermatitis, 66–73

Scales
Subacute eczematous dermatitis, 6, 7, 371
Psoriasis, 46–48
Seborrheic dermatitis, 66–73
Tinea corporis, 206–209

Lichenification
Chronic eczematous dermatitis, 6, 7, 371
Lichen simplex, 22, 23

Crusts
Any vesicular, eroded, excoriated, or ulcerated dermatitis

Vesicles
Scabies, 266–271
Acute eczematous dermatitis, 6, 7
Herpes zoster, 246

Ulcers
Syphilitic chancre, 254, 255

GENITALIA (MALE AND FEMALE)

Macules
Seborrheic dermatitis, 66–73
Secondary syphilis, 256, 257, 259
Vitiligo, 160–163

Papules or Plaques
Chronic eczematous dermatitis, 6, 7, 371
Psoriasis, 48, 49
Scabies, 266–271
Condylomata acuminata, 236, 237
Lichen planus, 96, 97
Secondary syphilis, 256, 257, 259
Melanoma, 386, 391

Nodules or Tumors
Squamous cell carcinoma, 336
Melanoma, 386, 391
Scabies (scrotum), 266

Vegetative Lesions
Condylomata acuminata, 236, 237
Condylomata lata, 236, 256, 259
Squamous cell carcinoma, 336

Lichenification
Chronic eczematous dermatitis, 6, 7, 371

Scales
Seborrheic dermatitis, 66–73
Moniliasis, 214–225
Psoriasis, 46, 47
Tinea cruris, 204, 205
Secondary syphilis, 256

Crusts (*see* Erosions; Ulcers; Vesicles)

Vesicles or Bullae
Acute eczematous dermatitis, 6, 7
Scabies, 266–271
Herpes simplex, 244
Erythema multiforme, 122–125

Pustules
Moniliasis, 214, 216, 217, 221, 223
Scabies, 266–271

Erosions
Herpes simplex, 244
Syphilitic chancre, 254, 255

Ulcers
Syphilitic chancre, 254, 255
Squamous cell carcinoma, 336

Excoriations
Scabies, 266–271

BUTTOCKS

Macules
Fixed-drug eruption, 42, 43

Papules
Scabies, 266–271

Wheals
Insect bites, 272, 273

Vesicles
Herpes simplex, 244
Scabies, 266–271
Tinea corporis, 206–209
Eczematous dermatitis, 6, 7, 371

Pustules
Tinea corporis, 206–209
Moniliasis, 214, 216
Scabies, 266–271

BUTTOCKS *(Cont.)*
  Scales
    Tinea corporis, 206–209
    Psoriasis, 46, 47

PERIANAL REGION
  Macules
    Seborrheic dermatitis, 66–73
    Tinea corporis, 206–209
  Papules or Plaques
    Chronic eczematous dermatitis,
      6–22
    Psoriasis, 46, 47
    Condylomata acuminata, 236, 237
    Condylomata lata, 256, 259
    Secondary syphilis, 256
  Vegetative Lesions
    Condylomata acuminata, 236, 237
    Condylomata lata (syphilis), 236,
      256, 259
  Scales
    Subacute eczematous dermatitis, 6–
      22
    Psoriasis, 46, 47
    Moniliasis, 214, 216
    Tinea corporis, 206–209
  Lichenification
    Chronic eczematous dermatitis
      (pruritus ani), 22, 23, 371
  Vesicles
    Acute eczematous dermatitis, 6, 7
  Erosions
    Moniliasis, 214, 216
    Syphilitic chancre, 254
  Fissures
    Psoriasis, 46, 47
    Chronic eczematous dermatitis, 22,
      23, 371
  Ulcers
    Syphilitic chancre, 254

ARMS AND FOREARMS
  Papules or Plaques
    Psoriasis, 46, 47, 55
    Lichen planus, 96, 97
    Lupus erythematosus, 134–139
    Chronic eczematous dermatitis,
      6–22, 371
    Melanocytic nevi, 288–299
  Nodules
    Melanoma, 386, 388–391

Carcinoma, squamous cell, 336
Granuloma annulare, 100, 101
  Scales
    Subacute or chronic eczematous
      dermatitis, 6–22, 371
    Psoriasis, 46, 47, 55
    Tinea corporis, 206–209
    Lupus erythematosus, 134–139
  Lichenification
    Chronic eczematous dermatitis, 22,
      23, 371
  Crusts
    Ecthyma, 176, 177

HANDS
  Macules
    Lentigo (dorsum), 286, 287
    Lupus erythematosus (dorsum),
      134–139
    Vitiligo (dorsum), 160–163
    Erythema multiforme, 122–125
    Secondary syphilis, 256, 257
  Papules or Plaques
    Subacute or chronic eczematous
      dermatitis, 6–22, 371
    Verruca vulgaris, 232, 233
    Verruca plana, 234, 235
    Solar keratosis (dorsum), 314, 315
    Scabies, 266–271
    Granuloma annulare, 100, 101
    Lupus erythematosus (dorsum),
      134–139
    Psoriasis, 46, 47, 58, 59, 62, 63
    Lichen planus, 96, 97
    Pyogenic granuloma (around nails),
      310, 311
    Erysipeloid, 188, 189
    Erythema multiforme (palm and dor-
      sum), 122–125
  Nodules or Tumors
    SKIN-COLORED
      Squamous cell carcinoma, 336,
        339
      Keratoacanthoma, 284, 285
      Verruca vulgaris, 232, 233
    ERYTHEMATOUS
      Granuloma annulare, 100, 101
      Pyogenic granuloma, 310, 311
    PIGMENTED
      Melanoma, 387, 391

Topographical Index of Differential Diagnosis   **403**

HANDS *(Cont.)*

Vegetative Lesions

Verruca vulgaris, 232, 233
Squamous cell carcinoma, 336–339
Keratoacanthoma, 284, 285

Scales

Subacute or chronic eczematous
dermatitis, 6–22, 371
Tinea manus, 202, 203
Psoriasis, 46, 47, 58, 59, 62, 63
Lupus erythematosus (dorsum),
134–139
Secondary syphilis, 256, 257

Hyperkeratosis

Solar keratosis (dorsum), 314, 315
Keratoacanthoma (dorsum), 284,
285
X-ray dermatitis, 316

Lichenification

Chronic eczematous dermatitis,
6–22, 371

Burrows

Scabies (between digits), 266–271

Vesicles or Bullae

Acute eczematous dermatitis, 6, 7
Dyshydrotic dermatitis, 26–29
Pompholyx (eczema), 26–29
Dermatophytosis, 202, 203
Scabies, 266–271
Porphyria (exposed areas), 142–148
Herpes simplex, 242
Erythema multiforme, 122–125

Pustules

Dermatophytosis, 202, 203
Eczematous dermatitis, 6–22, 371
Scabies, 266–271
Pustular psoriasis (palm) 60–62

Erosions

Moniliasis (webs of fingers),
214–216
Porphyria cutanea tarda, 142–145

Ulcers

Carcinoma, squamous cell, 336–339
Melanoma, 387–391
X-ray dermatitis, 316
Syphilitic chancre, 254

Scars

Porphyria cutanea tarda (discrete,
pink; on exposed areas),
142–145

FEET

Papules

Subacute or chronic eczematous
dermatitis, 6–22, 371
Verruca vulgaris (plantar region),
232
Secondary syphilis (plantar surface),
256, 257

Nodules or Tumors

Carcinoma, squamous cell, 336
Melanoma, 387–391

Scales

Tinea pedis (intertriginous areas particularly, 196–201
Subacute or chronic eczematous
dermatitis, 6–22, 371
Psoriasis, 58, 59

Vesicles

Tinea pedis, 196–201
Eczematous dermatitis. 6–22, 371
Pompholyx (eczema), 26–29

Lichenification

Chronic eczematous dermatitis,
6–22, 371

Vesicles or Bullae

Acute eczematous dermatitis, 6–22,
371
Tinea pedis, 196–201

Pustules

Pustular psoriasis, 62
Scabies, 266–271

Lichenification

Chronic eczematous dermatitis,
6–22, 371

Erosions

Tinea pedis, 196–201

LEGS

Papules or Plaques

Subacute or chronic eczematous
dermatitis, 6–22, 371
Psoriasis, 46, 47
Lichen planus, 96, 97
Ichthyosis, 166–169
Melanocytic nevi, 288–299

Vesicles or Bullae

Insect bites, 272–275
Eczematous dermatitis, 6–22, 371

Wheals

Insect bites, 272, 273

Subject Index

Recognize These Skin Alterations During the Routine Physical Examination*

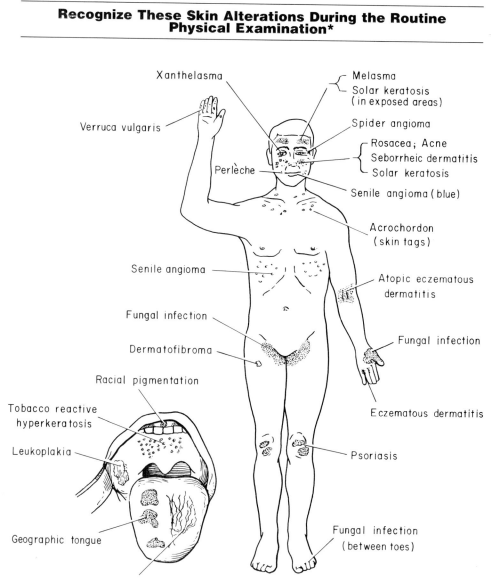

*From Fitzpatrick TB, Bernhard JD: The structure of skin lesions and fundamentals of diagnosis, in *Dermatology in General Medicine,* 3d ed. Edited by TB Fitzpatrick et al. New York, McGraw-Hill, 1987, pp 40–41.